To Jeanne and George Synan, the best mother- and father-in-law I could ever have asked for.
And to Kathy Felski: the best sister-in-law in the world.
—M.P.M.

For Mary, who fills my life with happiness.
—J.M.C.

Contents

Foreword

You have just opened a remarkable and practical book that could literally save your life. Research over the last 30 years has made it absolutely clear that high cholesterol is linked to heart disease and stroke. More than half of all Americans have higher-than-desirable cholesterol levels, and yet remarkably few ever actually do anything about it. One of the most important reasons for this is confusion: people simply don't know what to believe regarding cholesterol — and even if they believe it, they're not sure what to do. This issue recently became even more topical when one of the medications that lower cholesterol, Baycol, was withdrawn from the market worldwide because of several cases of severe muscle pain, some of which resulted in death. This event, which was widely publicized, has led many individuals to question the safety and wisdom of lowering cholesterol, particularly through taking medication. Yet all experts and virtually all doctors agree that lowering cholesterol is imperative for a large number of people, and can be lifesaving in many cases. Indeed, stroke is the most important cause of disability in the Western world, and heart disease remains by far the most common cause of death in the United States—and is rapidly on its way to becoming the most common cause of death worldwide. The risk of *both* these serious and life-threatening diseases can be markedly reduced when cholesterol is lowered. But until now, effective tools have been lacking for communicating the important information about how to lower cholesterol to the average person.

This book, *50 Ways to Lower Your Cholesterol*, is the most effective book on this topic that I have seen in my years of research and clinical practice in the field of cholesterol. Dr. Mary McGowan has teamed with her sister, Jo McGowan Chopra, to create a book consisting of practical, understandable advice about how to lower your cholesterol. Dr. McGowan has superb training and long experience in the treatment of people with high cholesterol, and her sister Jo brings a unique layperson's perspective to the writing of this book. So much about the cholesterol field has been confusing and controversial—from specific issues related to diet, such as the "fat versus carbohydrate" (Ornish versus Atkins) debate, to the use of supplements and alternative therapies to the safety of prescription medications. The authors of this book have skillfully explained all of the issues surrounding cholesterol in plain terms that can be clearly understood by persons who have no medical background. Medical and scientific issues are explained in an accurate yet understandable way, and advice is given that is applicable to all readers. The end result is a practical manual for lowering cholesterol that should be read by every adult who is concerned about their risk of developing heart disease or stroke, or who has already developed one of these problems. Dr. McGowan goes into careful detail about the withdrawal of the statin drug Baycol from the market. She explains that the events that precipitated this withdrawal were extremely rare and makes the key point that the risk of heart attack and stroke (from high cholesterol) is dramatically greater than any risk related to taking prescription medication for lowering cholesterol. Practical advice is given about how to minimize the risk of a serious complication when taking statin therapy.

Twenty chapters are devoted to the issue of diet and cholesterol. The authors don't advocate an extreme alteration in lifestyle; they understand that most people enjoy what they eat and want to eat healthfully without completely removing the pleasure from the culinary experience. For example, one tip involves a recipe for making french fries — one of the poster foods for unhealthful eating—actually healthy! The chapter on low-fat eating at ethnic restaurants taught me things I never knew. The final chapter in the section on diet discusses the complicated issue of alcohol and helps you make an informed decision.

The authors have included a comprehensive section on dietary supplements and other "alternative" approaches for lowering cholesterol. Interest in this area has exploded over the last decade, and is one of the most common topics that patients bring up with their doctors (many of whom are rather ignorant regarding the use of these items for cholesterol lowering and prevention of heart disease). The authors explain why the over-the-counter supplement Cholestin is effective. They discuss the use of margarines, such as

Benecol and Take Control, for lowering cholesterol. There's even a chapter on the Indian herb guggulipid, which is thought to have the ability to reduce cholesterol. Several chapters deal with the important issues of exercise and smoking cessation as they relate not only to cholesterol, but to overall cardiovascular fitness and prevention of heart disease and stroke.

The final section contains detailed information about each of the prescription cholesterol-lowering medications. This is the most comprehensive information that has been made available to the public, and it is delivered in practical, understandable terms. These chapters will be a tremendous resource for any patients who have been instructed by their doctor to take one of these medications, or who have heard about any of them and wish to learn more.

There's no question that readers of this book will come away with a markedly improved understanding about what cholesterol is and the role it plays in the development of heart disease and stroke, as well as the motivation to make changes in diet and lifestyle. As a cholesterol specialist who has spent years doing research and treating patients with cholesterol disorders, I was thrilled to read this book and feel for the first time that I have a scientifically accurate, understandable, and practical resource to which I can refer my patients and be confident that what they read reflects the best possible advice that an expert in this field could give a patient with high cholesterol.

Daniel J. Rader, M.D.

Acknowledgments

This book would never have come to be had it not been for the extraordinary patience of my husband, Tom, and my three children, Patrick, Liam, and Sheila.

For many people, medical school and residency are recalled as a grueling time, with too little sleep and too much intimidation. My own experience was quite the opposite. When I entered medical school at the University of Massachusetts, I encountered a group of physicians and teachers whose passion was teaching and whose goal was to make my fellow classmates and me good and caring doctors.

The seven years I spent at the University of Massachusetts Medical Center, first as a medical student and later as a resident physician, were challenging, exciting, and, yes, exhausting. There was so much to learn and so many people excited to teach. I am especially grateful to Drs. Joseph Alpert, Jim Dalen, Richard Irwin, Lou Braverman, Sarah Cheeseman, David Clive, Mel Pratter, Bruce Weinstein, Nelson Gantz, Abby Adams, Linda Pape, Joel Gore, Ira

Ockene, Fran Renzi, Sarah Stone and Donna Grogan, who taught me not only about illness but about health and motivation as well.

Many people remember the competition and cutthroat aspects of medical school. At the University of Massachusetts, it just did not occur; at least, I did not experience it. I know I learned as much from my classmates as from our teachers. The classmates, in turn, have become great physicians, teachers, and thinkers. I would like to thank my medical school classmates Drs. John Miller, Anne Cushing-Brescia, Beth Coates, Steven Rapaport, Jim Pellegrini, Seth Bilazarian, Elenie Chadbourne, Andy Coco, Michael Connolly, Elisabeth Haeger, Rawden Evans, Debbie Ehrenthal, Susan Lynch, Caroline Marten-Ellis, Bob Quirbach, Ina Ratner, Mary Ellen Taplin, Dan Sullivan, Kenny Colmer, Dan Carlucci, Kathy Fitzgerald, Ross Carol, Dennis Tighe, Mike Cohen, and Aaron Zuckerberg for their friendship and insights.

I would also like to thank my residency colleagues Wayne Hoover, Patty Soscia, Dan Carlucci, Joe Antaki, Denis Dupuis, Grace and Jim Desemone, Renee and Jim Doull, Doug Heller, Bernie Clifford, Martin Boucher, Steve Beaudette, Kristie Silver, Mary Ellen Taplin, Bob McGowen, Adrienne Withers-Bradley, Bob Clinton, David Rind, Sheila Kennedy, Karil Bellah, Michael Thompson, Paul Boffetti, Ron Caputo, Harvey and Allison Goldfine, Larry Greenwald, and Steve Beaudoin, for their insights and late-night discussions in the halls of U. Mass.

As I moved from the University of Massachusetts to Johns Hopkins Hospital, I continued to encounter wonderful teachers and mentors, including Drs. Peter Kwiterovich and Stephanie Kafonek. Because the field of lipid metabolism is rather small, I have been fortunate to remain in touch with both Peter and Stephanie. Over the last decade, both have continued to be a great source of encouragement.

When I left Johns Hopkins, I was lucky in taking a job at The New England Heart Institute, where our goal is to provide the best possible care to all patients. I would like to thank my partners—Beatty Hunter, Bob Dewey, Bill Bradley, Pat Lawrence, Connor Haugh, Bruce Hook, Brian Shea, Lou Fink, Michael Hearne, Gary Minkiewicz, Gerry Angoff, Steve Beaudette, Craig Berry, Peter Klemintowicz, Bill Graff, Mark Liebling, and David Goldberg, for recognizing that preventing a heart attack is as important as performing an angioplasty. The nurse practitioners and physician's assistants of the New England Heart Institute are also outstanding, including Jeanne Finn, Susan Horton, Judy Tsiorbas, David Allen, Jo-Anne Manson, Marilyn Daley, and Jacqueline Gannuscio.

As this book goes to press, Dr. Beatty Hunter is preparing to retire. During the decade we have worked together, I have been impressed not only with Beatty's intelligence, but his fairness and genuine kindness to staff, patients, and colleagues. I know I speak for the entire staff of the New England Heart Institute when I say Beatty will be missed tremendously.

My friends and colleagues at the Cholesterol Management Center make work a joy. Dr. Susan Lynch, my partner, is an expert on pediatric obesity and lipid disorders in children. Susan and I were lab partners in medical school and have been friends ever since. Mary Card, the best dietitian I have ever known, inspires everyone she meets — especially her patients—with her creativity and passion for nutrition and good food. Carolyn Finocchiaro, a gifted and wonderful nurse practitioner, has the perfect combination of gentleness, humor, and authority. Zena Ligon's talent for helping my patients relax makes their blood drawing painless, and Diane Hebert manages my schedule and my life with such dexterity that I move from one thing to another with never a hitch. Thanks also to Elizabeth, who keeps our hypertension clinical trials on track, and to Hope, Gail, and Lisa, who make it all happen. You are not only great colleagues but great friends as well.

Over the past decade I have also been fortunate to work with the members of the Northern New England Study Group—Drs. Bob Allen, Dave Malenka, Phil Ades, Len Keilson, Paul McGrath, Gerry O'Connor, David Charlesworth, Hebe Quinton, and John Raymond, who share my passion for cholesterol reduction.

I also consider myself extraordinarily lucky to be part of the "New England Group." Dr. Dick Pasternack spends a great deal of time bringing together some of the top people in the field of lipid metabolism for discussions and lively interchanges. The major meetings of the New England Lipid Group take place at Massachusetts General Hospital in Boston. These are open to anyone in the New England medical community. Periodically, Dr. Pasternack invites a smaller group together to plan future speakers for the group. As a result of these smaller meetings, I have opportunity to interact with some truly remarkable people. I have especially enjoyed getting to know Drs. Jorge Plutzky, Linda Cashin-Hemphill and Francie Welty.

In the last few years, I have also been truly blessed to have had the opportunity to get to know and learn from Drs. Dan Rader, Bill Castelli, Barry Effron, Roger Blumenthal, Wendy Post, Bob Lees, Ann Lees, Ishwarlal Jialal, Paul Thompson, Sid Alexander, and Evan Stein.

One of the most wonderful and brilliant men I have ever met was the late Dr. Roger Williams. Roger accomplished more in his short life then most people who are given twice as long. Even greater than Roger's contributions to the fields of lipid metabolism and cardiovascular genetics (which were many) were his tireless efforts on behalf of his patients. His death left the field with a major void. His friends, family and patients miss him tremendously.

Finally I must thank Susan Cohen, my literary agent, who suggested I do this project, and Ellen Vinz, an excellent editor who always found a nice way of pushing me along when I was slow in meeting deadlines.

Introduction

I hope you enjoy reading *50 Ways to Lower Your Cholesterol* as much as I enjoyed writing it. The suggestions I make in these pages are the same ones I follow myself. I not only feel good, but I enjoy the way my life feels.

Many things determine your cholesterol level: diet, weight, exercise, and genetics. The treatment of any cholesterol disorder, therefore, will usually require a multifaceted approach.

Diet, weight reduction, and initiation of an exercise plan require counseling and motivation. I find this aspect of my job extremely rewarding. If I can inspire my patients to improve their diet and begin an exercise program, I know that weight loss will follow. People who exercise regularly and eat a healthy, low-fat, well-balanced diet feel better, look better, and most importantly, lower their risk for heart disease and other chronic illnesses. You hear the old adage "You are what you eat!" so often. If you have made unsuccessful attempts to lower your cholesterol with diet and exercise in the past, this book is for you.

This book gives you the latest scientific information on nutritional supplements — why some work and others don't. If you choose to use supplements, it is important to know what to expect. How much will they lower your cholesterol? Are there side effects?

Finally, it is important to recognize that our genetics play a major role in determining our cholesterol levels. Two people can weigh the same amount, eat the same food, exercise an equal number of hours, and yet have radically different cholesterol levels. For most people with genetic cholesterol disorders or cardiac disease, diet, exercise, and supplements might improve things, but they are unlikely to fully correct the situation. These people will almost surely require medications to lower their cholesterol.

When it comes to taking cholesterol-lowering medications, many people worry about potential side effects (see page 53–54). Although I feel this is a very legitimate concern, it is important to know that in general, cholesterol-lowering medications are both extremely safe and very well tolerated by most people.

Recently, however, Baycol, a cholesterol-lowering medication in the statin family, was taken off the market. This prompted many of my patients, even those on other statins (such as Lipitor, Zocor, Mevacor, Pravachol, and Lescol), to become quite concerned. Many called me, asking if they should discontinue their statin. Since I feel strongly that the statins save lives, I of course took the time necessary to convince my patients to continue taking their statin medication. Here is the information I shared with my patients:

At the time Baycol was withdrawn from the market, about 11 million prescriptions had been written for this drug. Thirty-one people who took Baycol died of a disorder called rhabdomyolysis. This is a condition characterized by muscle-cell breakdown and eventual kidney failure. Most of the 31 people who died of rhabdomyolysis were also taking another medication, gemfibrozil (Lopid). (See chapter 48.) In 1999 Bayer, the company that made Baycol, warned doctors not to use Baycol and Lopid in combination. The company had determined that the Baycol/Lopid combination put people at increased risk for rhabdomyolysis. This is not surprising, since both of these medications have the potential to cause rhabdomyolysis independently of each other. Unfortunately, not all physicians were aware of this warning. Since Lopid has been successfully used in combination with other statins, it made more sense to take Baycol off the market than it did to remove Lopid.

Roughly half of all Americans die of heart disease or stroke. Statin medications have been shown to reduce the risk of developing a heart attack or stroke by roughly 30 to 48 percent. The risk of dying from rhabdomyolysis with Baycol, although low (31 deaths out of 11 million prescriptions), was higher than with any of the other available statins (Lipitor, Zocor, Mevacor, Pravachol, and Lescol).

Over the last three years, more than 300 million prescriptions have been written for these statins. In this time period, the Health Research Group reported 52 deaths related to rhabdomyolysis. This means that a person's chance of dying from rhabdomyolysis as a result of taking a statin is roughly 1 in 5,747,000 (1 in 5.7 million). There are many other medications that are associated with a much worse side-effect profile, and we take many of these medications without thinking twice. As noted by Dr. Alan Brown, a fellow lipid specialist: "The odds of a serious bleed from aspirin can be as high as 1 in 50,000."

No drug is without side effects. You should try to be as well-informed as possible regarding the side effects of the medications you are taking. In the case of the statins, the benefits clearly outweigh the risks.

You might ask if there are ways to reduce your risk of developing rhabdomyolysis while taking a statin. The answer is absolutely yes. If while on a statin, you develop total body muscle aches (like the way you feel just before coming down with the flu), call your doctor and get a CPK (muscle-enzyme blood level) test.

It is normal to have small amounts of muscle enzymes in your bloodstream. We all have a certain number of muscle cells that die on a daily basis. These cells release their enzymes into the bloodstream, where they can be measured. If you run a marathon, the level of muscle enzymes in your blood will become very high, but rapidly drops as your muscles recover. When a person begins taking a statin, we expect a small rise in the muscle enzymes. If the level rises significantly, we become concerned.

The CPK test is a simple blood test, and if it determines that your CPK is elevated, your physician will either take you off the statin or reduce the dose. In general, the muscle aches will disappear and your risk of rhabdomyolysis will diminish dramatically. The bottom line is, if you listen to your body you are likely to do beautifully on a statin.

Once the decision to use a medication has been made, your doctor must determine which medication is most appropriate and what dose you need. This book will help you determine which medication, if you decide to take one, might be best for you. Once you're armed with the proper medication information, you will be able to have a meaningful discussion with your personal physician.

If you are already on medication but your cholesterol levels remain high (or your protective cholesterol remains low), it is important not to get discouraged. Over the next few years there will be an explosion of new therapies available for the treatment of cholesterol disorders. At the New England Heart Institute, where I work, we are currently working with many new medications. This book will give you an idea of what new medications are on the horizon.

No matter what your cholesterol disorder is, there is hope. This book will give you the tools you need to normalize your cholesterol levels. If high cholesterol and heart disease run in your family, you can make changes that will dramatically reduce your risk of a heart attack. In essence, you can change your destiny.

I have worked in the field of cholesterol metabolism for over a decade, and I can honestly say that I have met very few people whose cholesterol levels I have not been able to normalize. Actually, I don't normalize my patients' cholesterol profiles; they do it themselves. My job is to be a good teacher and a tireless (or tiresome, depending on your mood!) motivator. It is not enough for me to be an expert in the field of cholesterol metabolism. I might understand all the intricacies of how cholesterol is produced and metabolized, but if I don't understand the people who are doing the metabolizing, I can't help them succeed.

When I meet a person who has a cholesterol problem, I need to know who she is. I want to know how she spends her time. Does she travel for work, or does she work at home? Is she retired, or busy with small children? And what about her leisure time? Does she enjoy active sports, or is she more likely to spend her free time reading, going to movies, in front of the computer, or dining out?

It is also crucial for me to know with whom my patient lives. Are the people at home going to help or hinder you? Could they benefit from cholesterol reduction too? It is essential for me to know what foods a person grew up eating and what his current diet consists of. I need to know what a person's favorite foods are. I ask about exercise; I want to know how frequently he exercises and how long each session lasts. If he has a regular exercise program, I want to know if it is a new program or something he has been doing for years.

Smoking can alter cholesterol quite dramatically, so I need to know about smoking history. And because certain illnesses and chronic medical conditions and medications can affect cholesterol, it is important for me to know a person's entire medical history. Cholesterol abnormalities are often genetic in nature; therefore I always inquire about a family history of high cholesterol and heart disease.

My first visit with a new patient takes about an hour and forty-five minutes. (Forty-five minutes with registered dietician Mary Card and one hour with me.) The information I obtain during our first visit helps me understand who a person is. Even if two people have identical cholesterol profiles, if one of them is a 45-year-old traveling salesperson who is on the road five days a week and has three teenage children at home, and the other is a 75-year-old retired schoolteacher who lives alone and has had a bypass, my diet and exercise recommendations — and even my medication choices — are likely to be radically different.

Finally, I always ask my patients how motivated they are to get their cholesterol under control. Generally, the more motivated a person is, the more successful he or she is.

Unless you come to see me in my office at the New England Heart Institute, I am unlikely to have the benefit of meeting you personally. But even without a face-to-face meeting, this book will be able to guide you through the steps necessary to dramatically improve your cholesterol profile. I will give you estimates regarding how much a certain lifestyle change or medication is likely to benefit your cholesterol.

Of course, not everything in the book will pertain to you. For example, you might have very high triglycerides and a normal LDL cholesterol level. You will obviously be much more interested in the information on triglyceride reduction. Likewise, if you don't smoke and never have, you can skip over the information on the effects of quitting smoking on cholesterol. I have tried to write this book in an easy-to-read, conversational style, so even if some of the information doesn't pertain to you, it might be fun to read. Then you will be able to offer advice to your friends and family, if they smoke or have cholesterol problems different from yours.

PART ONE

What Is Cholesterol?

I remember when a cholesterol level of 300 mg/dl was considered normal. How could this be? So-called "normal" laboratory values are determined by sampling a large number of people, tossing out the very highest and lowest lab values, and calling the range of values in between "normal." In a country where every year, 1.5 million people suffer a heart attack and another five hundred thousand die of heart disease, "normal" may not be desirable.

In 1948 the Framingham Heart Study, an ambitious study undertaken by the National Heart Institute (now known as the National Heart, Lung, and Blood Institute) examined the causes of cardiovascular disease. Their research taught us that an elevated cholesterol level is a strong risk factor for the development of a cardiac event (angina, heart attack, bypass surgery, or angioplasty).

What exactly is cholesterol? Why do we have it in our blood? And if the old "normal" cholesterol level is too high, what blood level is safe and acceptable?

Cholesterol is a white, waxy substance that is found in some of the foods we eat; it is also manufactured by all the cells of our body, but most notably by the liver cells. Some cholesterol is essential to good health. Not only is cholesterol an important component of cell walls, it is also essential for the production of certain hormones. For most people, between 70 and 75 percent of the cholesterol in their blood is manufactured by their liver; the other 25 to 30 percent comes from the food they eat.

A person can have an elevated cholesterol level for a variety of reasons. There are a number of genetic abnormalities that result either in a dramatic increase in the liver's production of cholesterol or a decrease in the liver's ability to clear cholesterol from the blood. Certain diseases are associated with cholesterol elevations. These include diabetes and kidney, liver, and thyroid disease. Some medications cause cholesterol elevations. Finally, for many people, a diet rich in fat, calories, and cholesterol is the culprit.

When it comes to diet, fat and calories (not dietary cholesterol) are the worst offenders. When a person consumes excess fat, the liver becomes less efficient at removing cholesterol from the blood. And for many people, excess calories result in the overproduction of cholesterol by the liver. Dietary cholesterol has some impact on a person's cholesterol level, but there is a cap. For example, if a person who typically consumes about 100 mg of cholesterol per day increases his intake to about 400 mg per day, he can expect a dramatic increase in blood cholesterol. (For some people the increase can be as much as 60 mg/dl.) If this same person now jumps from 400 to 1,000 mg of cholesterol per day (the equivalent of adding about two egg yolks), his cholesterol will not rise any further. This "ceiling" effect is the reason that some people claim that eggs have no impact on their cholesterol. They were already above the ceiling of 400 mg per day. In our clinic we focus primarily on fat. However because fat and cholesterol typically come packaged together, our diet generally limits people to about 100 mg of dietary cholesterol.

In order to determine if your cholesterol level puts you at risk for the development of heart disease, you need to have your cholesterol level measured. In order to accurately measure your blood cholesterol level, you must fast for 12 hours prior to the test. Although it is certainly possible to measure the cholesterol when a person is not fasting, doctors can obtain a more complete picture of your cholesterol profile when you are in the fasting state. Once you have the results of your cholesterol tests back, you can use Table 1 to determine if you have a problem with any of the blood fats:

TABLE 1 Desirable Levels of Blood Fats

Blood Fat	*Desirable Level*
Total cholesterol	< 200 mg/dl (if no CAD*) < 150 mg/dl (if CAD)
Triglycerides	< 150 mg/dl (if no CAD) < 100 mg/dl (if CAD)
LDL cholesterol	< 130 mg/dl (if no CAD) < 100 mg/dl (if CAD) Ideal < 80 mg/dl (if CAD)
HDL cholesterol	> 45 mg/dl

*CAD = Coronary Artery Disease (generally defined as having had a heart attack, bypass, angioplasty, or having had an abnormal stress test indicating heart disease.) Diabetes also dramatically increases the risk of developing a cardiac event. If you have diabetes, your cholesterol goals are the same as a person who has CAD.

The total cholesterol is really the composite of many substances, including the triglycerides, LDL cholesterol, and HDL cholesterol. The triglycerides are blood fats that tend to rise in the face of alcohol intake, increased weight, a diet rich in sugar and fat, and a sedentary lifestyle. There is no doubt that elevated triglycerides increase the risk of developing heart disease and stroke. It has been shown that people who have high triglycerides also tend to have elevations in blood pressure and increased risk for developing diabetes.

It follows that the way to lower your triglycerides is to cut back on alcohol, exercise daily, restrict sugar and fat in your diet, and lose weight if necessary. For some people, the addition to the diet of high doses of fish oil will markedly lower triglycerides. Ensuing chapters outline the specifics of how to lower your triglycerides with lifestyle changes.

Sometimes, however, lifestyle changes alone are inadequate. If this proves true in your case, your doctor may prescribe a triglyceride-lowering medication such as Tricor, Lopid, or Niaspan.

LDL cholesterol stands for low-density lipoprotein cholesterol. You have probably heard of the "good and bad cholesterol." LDL cholesterol is the "bad cholesterol." Elevated levels of LDL cholesterol dramatically increase a person's risk for heart disease and stroke. LDL cholesterol sticks to the artery wall and over time can cause artery blockages to develop.

Most people who have a heart attack do not have a complete cholesterol blockage of the heart artery when the attack occurs. The cholesterol plaque (blockage), which contains large amounts of LDL cholesterol, can become unstable. This may cause the plaque to crack open. When this happens, the body's natural response is to try to repair the area with a blood clot. The combination of a ruptured cholesterol plaque and a blood clot can spell disaster. If the artery is totally blocked, a heart attack will occur.

If LDL cholesterol is a problem for you, it will be important to restrict dietary fat (especially saturated and hydrogenated fats). Likewise, if you need to lose weight, doing so will help lower the LDL cholesterol. Exercise has a modest role in LDL reduction. Specific dietary maneuvers, such as the addition of the plant stanol or sterol margarines (Benecol Light and Take Control, respectively), soy protein, flaxseed, fiber, psyllium, walnuts, or guggulipid (an Indian herb), can dramatically improve some people's cholesterol profiles.

Finally, if these measures fail, your doctor may prescribe one of the "statin" medications: Lipitor (atorvastatin), Zocor (simvastatin), Mevacor (lovastatin), Lescol (fluvastatin), or Pravachol (pravastatin). Niaspan (niacin), Welchol (colesevelam), and Tricor (fenofibrate) also lower LDL. For people who shun prescription medications, Cholestin is an over-the-counter product that is very similar to Mevacor. Likewise, there are many over-the-counter niacin preparations. In addition to the medications just listed, there are many new agents in various stages of development. Our team is now working with a medication that lowers LDL by as much as 70 percent. By the time you have finished this book, you will be armed with all the material you need to markedly reduce your LDL level.

The HDL cholesterol (high-density lipoprotein cholesterol) is also known as "good cholesterol." The role of HDL cholesterol is to bring the bad cholesterol back to the liver for processing. People with high levels of this type of cholesterol appear to be partially protected from heart disease. Of course, a person can have an excellent HDL cholesterol level and still develop heart disease. These people tend to have several other risk factors, such as high blood pressure, diabetes, and cigarette smoking. In large part, a person's HDL cholesterol level is genetically predetermined (meaning your level really depends on the genes your parents have given you). There are, however, some things you can do to improve your HDL cholesterol level. Quitting smoking can increase your HDL cholesterol level by as much as 8 mg/dl. Generally, the full impact is seen within six months of quitting.

Exercise is also known to improve HDL cholesterol. Men tend to get a greater increase in HDL cholesterol during the first year of exercise (as much as 10 percent), but if women keep at it, studies have shown as much as a 20-percent improvement over a five-year period. Men can maintain their 10-percent improvement with continued exercise but rarely experience further benefit over time. Weight loss can lead to a significant improvement in this lipoprotein, but often as a person is actively losing weight the HDL cholesterol level will decline transiently. Don't get discouraged if this happens to you. Once you reach a new weight plateau, your HDL level will increase and ultimately will exceed your old level.

Diet, too, can have an impact on HDL. People who eat high-fat, processed foods, such as commercially prepared baked goods (cookies, muffins, donuts) or deep-fried foods such as French fries, fried dough, and fried fish, take in large quantities of trans fat, a form of fat known to dramatically lower HDL. For these people, switching to monounsaturated fats—like the ones found in canola, olive, and peanut oils—can improve HDL levels. These people may also benefit from using avocados, walnuts, peanuts, almonds, filberts, or pistachios as a fat source. Finally, if you require more HDL improvement than the aforementioned measures can provide, your doctor may prescribe Niaspan, Lopid, or Tricor.

Unfortunately, many people with low HDL levels fail to fully normalize their level despite making lifestyle changes or using medication. A number of companies are looking at novel ways to improve the HDL level. Strategies include intravenous medications, the development of particles that mimic HDL activity, and even gene therapy. It is my opinion that within the next five years we will have dramatically improved methods of treating people with low HDL.

Once you have determined that you have a problem with cholesterol, it is important to determine the cause and develop a plan for improving your cholesterol level. Failure to do so may result in a heart attack, stroke, or even death.

There are a number of well-described genetic cholesterol abnormalities that result in markedly elevated triglycerides and/or LDL cholesterol levels. For example, some people have a genetic problem called familial hypercholesterolemia; these people—despite an outstanding diet, regular exercise, and maximum doses of cholesterol-lowering medications—will still have uncontrollable cholesterol levels. In these cases, LDL apheresis may be lifesaving. This dialysis-like procedure filters LDL cholesterol out of a person's blood, resulting in as much as a 70 to 80 percent reduction in the LDL level. The effect is, however, temporary. As a result, LDL apheresis must be performed twice a month.

Still other genetic disorders result in a tremendous reduction in the HDL level. Each of these disorders has the
potential to substantially increase cardiac risk.

Often an underlying illness or disease state will result in
a significant cholesterol abnormality. People with adult-
onset diabetes tend to have elevated triglycerides, depressed
HDL, and moderately elevated LDL levels. It has been my
experience that until blood sugar is under good control, it
is impossible to normalize the triglycerides in a person with
diabetes.

People with both underactive and overactive thyroid
glands can have a variety of cholesterol abnormalities. Thyroid disorders are much more common in women than men.
I have found that occasionally, correcting the underlying
thyroid disorder results in full normalization of the cholesterol profile, but more commonly the cholesterol profile
improves slightly but still needs work.

Nephrotic syndrome is a kidney disorder characterized
by large amounts of protein in the affected person's urine.
The body responds to this loss of protein by increasing the
amount of protein produced in the liver (in an attempt to
correct the blood protein level). Proteins carry blood
cholesterol; therefore it is not surprising to see a rise in
cholesterol level in this situation. Similarly, liver disease can
result in the overproduction of lipoproteins (blood fats).

Medication and Cholesterol

As your physician works with you to lower your cholesterol
level, she must carefully assess your medications. Some
medications can lead to alterations in blood cholesterol

levels. Table 2 reviews the effects of some commonly used medications:

TABLE 2 The Effects of Medication on Cholesterol Levels

	Triglycerides	*LDL*	*HDL*
Amiodarone	increase	increase	no significant change
Androgens	may increase	increase	reduction
Beta-blockers	increase	no significant change	reduction
Cyclosporin	increase	increase	no significant change
Progestins	no significant change	increase	reduction
Protease Inhibitors	increase	may increase	no significant change
Retinoids	increase	increase	reduction
Steroids	increase	increase	increase
Diuretics	increase	increase	no significant change

You may wonder what some of these medications are or how they are used. Amiodorone (Cordarone, Pacerone) is used in the treatment of certain heart arrhythmias. Androgens, such as Android capsules or Testoderm, are used frequently in the treatment of males with testosterone insufficiency or in the treatment of certain cancers in women.

Beta-blockers are blood pressure medications. Not all beta-blockers adversely impact cholesterol. Acebutolol (Sectral), carteolol (Cartrol), carvedilol (Coreg), celiprolol (Selectrol), penbutolol (Levatol), and pindolol (Visken) are the beta-blockers that generally do not have an adverse impact on lipids. On the other hand, the most commonly used beta-blockers—including atenolol (Tenormin), metoprolol (Lopressor, Toprol), nadolol (Corgard), and propranolol (Inderal)—all adversely affect blood lipid levels. However, the beta-blockers with an adverse impact are actually the group of beta-blockers shown to protect against recurrent heart attack in people who have already suffered one. For this reason, it is sometimes essential to use a beta-blocker and work around the adverse impact on lipids.

Cyclosporin (Neoral, Sandimmune) is an immunosuppressive agent and is used in people who have undergone a heart or kidney transplant. For these people the drug is irreplaceable, and its impact on blood lipids must be dealt with.

Progestins are one of the components of most birth control pills and are used as part of postmenopausal hormone-replacement therapy. In general, the goal is to use the lowest possible dose of a progestin. In the case of birth control pills, the agents that have the least negative impact on the cholesterol profile include Ortho Tri-Cyclen, Modicon, and Brevicon. When progestins (such as Cycrin, Provera, or Prometrium capsules) are used as part of the postmenopausal hormone regime, the goal is to use the lowest possible dose. In the Postmenopausal Estrogen Progestin Intervention (PEPI) Trial, the progestin with the least negative impact on the lipoprotein profile was micronized progestin. (Prometrium is an example of micronized progestin.) Protease inhibitors—such as Crixivan, Agenerase capsules, Fortovase, Invirase, Norvir, and Viracept—have dramatically improved the lives of people with HIV/AIDS, but like most things, they come with a price. People on the protease inhibitors experience a marked increase in blood lipids, most notably a dramatic increase in triglycerides. For most people, the protease inhibitors simply cannot be discontinued. In general, people on these agents require a lipid-altering agent. Because both protease inhibitors and lipid-altering medications can adversely impact liver function, it is crucial to follow, very closely, patients taking both agents.

Retinoids, such as Accutane, are used in the treatment of cystic acne. Thankfully, most people on Accutane are teenagers who use it for brief periods of time. Although lipids can be dramatically and adversely altered with Accutane, levels typically revert to normal following therapy.

Steroids, such as prednisone, are frequently used for short periods in the treatment of poison ivy or for an attack of asthma. If a person's asthma attacks, or exposure to poison ivy, are infrequent, the negative impact on the lipid profile presents little worry. Unfortunately, there are many people on chronic steroids for a host of rheumatologic disorders, severe asthma, chronic lung disorders, or to prevent rejection of transplanted organs. For these people, the adverse impact on lipids will require careful management. It is crucial to expose patients who will require lifelong steroids to the lowest possible dose. In some cases it is possible to use steroid-sparing medications (medications that will allow the use of a lower dose of a steroid) along with the steroid itself.

Finally, diuretics, another type of medication used to lower blood pressure, can markedly alter the cholesterol profile. Again, in some cases, they are absolutely necessary. It should be remembered that indapamide (Lozol) is one diuretic that has very little negative impact on cholesterol levels.

If one of the medications mentioned appears to be the culprit in your high cholesterol, your doctor may want to alter
your medications in hopes of improving your cholesterol.
The chapters that follow will guide you through the steps
necessary to fully normalize your cholesterol level. Diet,
exercise, and the proper supplements will do the trick for
many people. However, if your cholesterol remains stubbornly high despite your best efforts at diet and exercise,
don't be afraid to take a medication. Cholesterol-lowering
medications are among the best-studied drugs on the planet.
While some people may develop side effects, the vast major-
ity do not. If your physician follows your case closely, it is
highly unlikely that you will ever have a problem.

PART TWO

Diet

1. Watch Your Cholesterol Consumption

Keep your cholesterol consumption at or below 100 milligrams per day. There is no need to count milligrams of cholesterol, as you will by necessity keep the level low simply by restricting fat and eliminating whole eggs from your diet. Cholesterol is found only in products of animal origin. For example, meat, poultry, fish, cheese, eggs, and milk all contain cholesterol, while cooking oils (even palm oil and coconut oil) do not.

If you don't like the look of a very small piece of meat on your plate, try "stretching" your meat serving by incorporating it into a vegetable-rich stir-fry. Ideal choices for stir-frying include chicken, shrimp, scallops, and lamb. You can save on fat and calories while stir-frying by using cooking spray instead of oil. Cooking sprays come in a variety of flavors, including garlic, olive oil, and butter. The stir-fry can be served on rice.

2. Be Smart About Carbohydrates

These days many people worry about carbohydrates. In fact, eliminating them has become a very popular diet strategy. But you shouldn't think that rice or potatoes make you fat; they don't. Of course, like any foods, they can cause problems when they are consumed in excess. Rice and potatoes don't contain any fat to speak of, but they do contain calories.

So what constitutes a serving of rice? Answer: Half a cup of cooked rice. Unfortunately, many people go overboard on both rice and potatoes. Our patients are often shocked when we show them a food model. Most people consume one and one-half to two cups of rice and eat a potato twice the size we typically recommend. Once you are clear on what a portion is and you stick with it, rice and potatoes can be your friends. Try to purchase brown rice, as it is more nutrient-rich than white.

3. Lower Your Sugar Intake

As you aim to lower your cholesterol, it is not just fat and calories that matter; sugar can also be very problematic. I often see patients who are sent to me because they "failed" a low-fat diet. Often their doctor has told them that their cholesterol is high and that they should cut back on fat. If they are lucky, the doctor might spend a few minutes more pointing out the foods that are notoriously high in fat (red meat, whole milk, cheese), but that is all the information patients receive.

It is hard to blame physicians for spending so little time. First of all, we get very little nutrition education in medical school. Secondly, many doctors are very pressed for time; a typical visit lasts only about 15 minutes—hardly enough time to deliver worthwhile dietary advice. Patients, then, are pretty much left on their own to figure out what constitutes a low-fat diet. Many people try to cut out all fat. This is impossible because even vegetables have a trace amount of fat.

In the quest to completely eliminate fat, many people make substitutions. In some cases, substitutions are excellent choices (replace butter with either Benecol Light or diet margarine, replace red meat with chicken or fish). In other situations, the replacement may be low in fat but extraordinarily high in sugar. And a high-sugar diet not only markedly increases triglycerides; it has lots of calories as well.

Because having high triglycerides appears to significantly increase the risk for heart disease, lowering an elevated triglyceride level is crucial. Interestingly, studies have shown that an elevated triglyceride level may portend the development of diabetes. A person may have an elevated triglyceride level for years before he or she develops diabetes.

4. Maintain Your Ideal Weight

People who come to see us for the first time often want to know exactly how much fat they eat in a day. They also want to know how much they should weigh. Although the answer differs for each person, here are a few basic guidelines.

Many people who come to see us not only need to lower their cholesterol, they need to lose weight as well. We find that most women lower their cholesterol and lose weight on a diet containing between 27 and 30 grams of fat and 1,200 calories per day. Most men do the same on between 35 and 40 grams of fat and 1,500 calories per day.

In our program, we tend to use something called the body mass index, or BMI, to assess a person's weight. The BMI requires measurement of weight in kilograms and height in meters; because it is unlikely that you think in kilograms or meters, I suggest you use Table 3:

TABLE 3 Ideal Weight for Men and Women

	Men	**Women**
First 5 feet of height	105 lbs.	100 lbs.
For every inch over 5 feet add	6 lbs.	5 lbs.

For example, a woman who is 5 feet 6 inches tall should weigh 130 lbs. A man who is 5 feet 10 inches tall should weigh 165. Obviously, there is a range for weight. Some people do have a larger frame than others.

One of the things I tell people the first time I meet them is that I will not take away their "occasion dinners." An "occasion dinner" might be a birthday or an anniversary dinner where a person goes out to the best restaurant in town and neither looks at price nor thinks about calories. Occasion dinners, by definition, happen *occasionally*. (Of course, we have a problem if you have a very big family and you find yourself celebrating five or six times a month.) Rather than focusing on these big and obvious splurges, I ask people to concentrate on their daily habits.

5. Switch to Whole-Grain Cereal for Breakfast

Often people admit that they might occasionally have a low-fat muffin or deli-style bagel for breakfast. If this is your situation, it is important for you to know that a low-fat muffin may contain as many as 15 teaspoons of sugar and 400 calories. A deli-style bagel may be very low in fat, but it also contains a whopping 400 to 450 calories—and that is before the cream cheese.

From the point of view of your cholesterol, your weight, your heart, and even your wallet, you are much better off eating breakfast at home. Great breakfast choices include a bowl of whole-grain cereal (Wheaties, Total, Cheerios, oatmeal, Bran Buds or Grape Nuts) with skim or 1 percent low-fat milk, or a whole-wheat English muffin with Benecol Light. (Benecol is a plant stanol margarine that really does lower cholesterol. In fact, Benecol can lower LDL by as much as 14 percent. I will review this margarine in detail in chapter 23.) On weekends, try an Egg Beater omelet loaded with vegetables, whole-grain toast, Benecol Light, and soy breakfast sausages.

6. Cut Back on Cream and Sugar in Your Coffee

What do you eat for breakfast? If you are like many of my patients, your answer may be, "I don't eat breakfast." My response is, "Not even coffee?" The typical answer is, "Well, of course I have coffee; I pick it up at the drive-through on my way to work." Then I ask how they take their coffee.

Many people ask for their coffee "regular." A regular cup of coffee can have as many as 250 calories (due to cream and sugar). If you have ever watched a regular cup of coffee being prepared, you know as well as I that the cream nozzle stays open for a good long while, and the sugar is certainly not measured in level teaspoons. There are many of you reading this who might consume several of these "regular" cups of coffee a day. You may wonder why you can't lower your cholesterol or why it is so hard to lose weight.

Even if you only get rid of the cream and switch to whole milk in your coffee, you will see a difference. Over time, your goal should be to drink your coffee black or with skim milk. An alternative is fat-free half-and-half, which tastes great and adds no fat and very few calories to your coffee. You might try buying the fat-free half-and-half and a travel mug. You will save a great deal of money and will lower your cholesterol by making the coffee at home, using the fat-free half-and-half, and using the travel mug for your commute to work. You may even save time because the lines are often very long for coffee in the morning.

You should also try to get rid of the sugar in your coffee. Sugar, like cream, has lots of calories. In a country where 61 percent of the adult population is overweight or obese, the last thing we need is more calories. If you need your coffee to taste sweet, try a sugar substitute. Although I personally think it is wise to try to limit the use of sugar substitutes, moderate use does not appear to be harmful.

7. Pay Attention to Portion Size

As you settle down to dinner, the most important thing to think about is portion size. Many people eat all the right foods but still don't lose weight or fully normalize their cholesterol level. This is because they eat *too much* of the right foods.

Consider having a cup of clear broth soup before dinner. Soup is eaten by the spoonful; this will slow you down and hopefully fill you up. If you make or purchase a more hearty soup, it can become a main course. I love soup and frequently make a minestrone or meatless bean chili. When served with a whole-grain bread and/or salad, there is no need to eat anything more.

If you expect to lower your cholesterol level, it is important to reevaluate the space on your plate. Vegetables must take up most of it. To prevent boredom, it is important to incorporate a wide variety of vegetables into your evening meal. I am amazed by the number of people who limit themselves to peas, corn, carrots, and green beans. What about acorn squash, asparagus, artichokes, beets, broccoli, brussels sprouts, cauliflower, eggplant, kale, mushrooms, onions, parsnips, peppers, potatoes, radishes, summer squash, turnip, and zucchini? These are the things that you should be filling up on.

Meat should be served in very small portions (no more than four to six ounces). Red meat (which includes pork, beef, and ham) should be eaten only once (at the most, twice) a week. Chicken, turkey, and fish (snapper, perch, sole, cod, and halibut) are all good choices. Fatty fish, such as salmon and sardines, appears to confer some special heart-protecting benefits and should be consumed at least twice a week. Shellfish (oysters, scallops, clams, shrimp, lobster, crab) can be eaten on a near-daily basis. Many people are surprised when I tell them shellfish is a great choice. Having heard that shellfish contains a fair amount of cholesterol, many people feel that it is off-limits. In fact, shellfish contains far less cholesterol and dramatically less fat than red meat. Oysters, scallops, and clams contain less cholesterol than shrimp, lobster, and crab.

8. Vary Fruits and Vegetables in Your Diet

One of the things I find most interesting about diet (and it is true in my own family as well) is that most of us eat the same things over and over every day. Think about it. I bet you essentially eat the same breakfast and lunch at least Monday through Friday. For dinner, studies have shown that most American families cook from the same eight or nine recipes week in week out.

If you are going to eat the same things over and over, you need to make sure that the choices you are making for yourself and your family are low in fat, rich in nutrients, and high in taste. Even if you basically eat the same meals week in, week out, I do think you should try to vary the fruits and vegetables. This allows you to take in a wide variety of nutrients.

9. Make Those French Fries Healthy

If you have a little time and want to make French fries to go with your meal, try this easy recipe. Wash a few potatoes, peel them, and slice as you would French fries. Spray a nonstick cookie sheet with cooking spray and place the potato slices on the sheet. Coat slices with cooking spray, sprinkle with salt, and place them in the oven at 350 degrees for about 25 to 30 minutes (turning the fries occasionally). Turn the oven up to broil just until the French fries become golden-brown.

My children love these and so do their neighborhood friends. We live in a small town where everyone knows what I do for a living, so it is sometimes embarrassing when my kids loudly ask (in the local supermarket) if they can have hot dogs and fries for supper. What those who might hear them don't know is that my kids love Smart Dogs (a soy hot dog) and my French fries. When served with fresh vegetables (carrot slices, cucumber, grape tomatoes, red and yellow pepper), the meal is a great, low-fat, nutrient-rich choice.

10. Cut Out Regular Mayonnaise

Many people proudly tell me that they have a tuna sandwich for lunch nearly every day. If the sandwich is made using low-fat or nonfat mayonnaise, it is a great choice; but if the sandwich is made using regular mayonnaise (as it is at a deli or typical restaurant), it will generally contain 30 to 32 grams of fat.

11. Eat a Healthy Lunch

If you are in the habit of bringing your lunch to work or have the luxury of eating at home, there are lots of good low-fat options. How about a turkey, tuna, or chicken sandwich on whole grain or Lavash bread, prepared with mustard, low-fat mayonnaise, or Benecol Light? A peanut-butter sandwich can easily be worked in, but you should limit the peanut butter to a couple of teaspoons. You might think about having a low-fat, low-calorie TV dinner. Our clinic favors the Healthy Choice, Lean Cuisine, or Weight Watchers varieties.

Soup—either homemade or store-bought—makes a great lunch. As you look for a low-fat soup, you should also consider the fiber content. Soups with beans contain water-soluble fiber, which has been shown to lower cholesterol. Many brands of low-fat, high-fiber soups are available: some canned, some in cups to which boiling water is added.

Another great lunch (or supper) choice is a soy burger or soy hot dog. These can be prepared in the microwave and are loaded with both soy protein and fiber.

Lunch is a great time to fit in a piece of fruit. Varying your fruit choices will provide you with a host of different vitamins and minerals and will prevent boredom. Try to branch out beyond the traditional apple, orange, or banana. These are excellent choices, but apricots, cherries, nectarines, grapes, plums, peaches, star fruit, ugli fruit, blueberries, melon, strawberries, and kiwi can make your lunch a little more interesting.

Many people feel that a sandwich is not a sandwich without a bag of potato chips. Instead of regular chips, try baked chips or pretzels. And if you simply have to end your lunch with a sweet treat, consider having a cup of hot cocoa made with skim milk and a couple of graham crackers, flavored popcorn cakes (in my house caramel and chocolate are very popular), or animal crackers. If you are eating at home, a sugar-free Fudgsicle or Creamsicle is a low-fat, low-calorie choice.

12. Make Sure That Salad Really Is Healthy

If you are trying to lose weight and lower your cholesterol, you might choose a salad at either lunch or supper. A salad topped with grilled chicken or shrimp can be an excellent choice, but you need to be aware that using regular (full-fat) salad dressing can totally defeat the purpose. I remember a patient being so disappointed when his cholesterol level didn't budge after he gave up his daily roast-beef sandwich. He had replaced it by alternating a Greek salad with a Caesar salad every day for three months. He was shocked to find that the feta cheese and Greek dressing probably contained about 30 to 40 grams of fat, not to mention the gram of fat contained in each olive. . . And even though olives contain primarily monounsaturated fat, they still have calories. The Caesar salad also contains about 40 grams of fat. This time the culprits are the croutons, Parmesan cheese, and dressing. You can, however, reduce the fat dramatically by asking for both the cheese and dressings on the side. Sprinkle a teaspoon of cheese on your salad; you will get the flavor without a lot of fat. And if you dip your fork in the dressing and then spear your greens, you will get the flavor of the dressing with a fraction of the fat.

The things that make an innocent salad into a high-fat, high-calorie choice are croutons, regular dressings, and mayonnaise-based additions (chicken, tuna, pasta). There are plenty of excellent fat-free croutons and salad dressings. And if you like the idea of adding a mayonnaise-based salad to your greens, use a fat-free or low-fat mayonnaise.

Most supermarkets have a salad bar where you can create your own fresh salad and pay by the pound. It is also easy to buy the ingredients and make a nutrient-rich salad at home. As you prepare your salad, be daring. Expand your horizons beyond the traditional iceberg lettuce, hothouse tomatoes, and cucumber. A salad can be a complete meal.

Start out with dark greens; these are often called spring greens and frequently come prewashed. The darker the greens, the more nutrient-rich they are. Washed spinach can be an excellent choice too. Add carrots; blanched broccoli or cauliflower; grape tomatoes; mushrooms; and red, yellow, and orange peppers. Small amounts of chopped almonds or walnuts can add crunch to your salad. Salads are also a great place to add garbanzo beans (chickpeas). Sometimes raisins or tangerines make a great addition to a salad. Topping the salad with small amounts of grilled chicken, tuna, or swordfish can turn the salad into your main meal.

13. Avoid Fast Food

Fast food is a big player at lunchtime. Table 4 reviews the fat and calorie content of many fast-food favorites:

TABLE 4 Calorie, Fat, and Sodium Content of Fast Foods

	Calories	Fat (g)	Sodium (mg)
BOSTON MARKET			
Skinless Turkey Breast (5 oz)	170	1	850
¼ White Chicken Breast (no skin) (4.5 oz)	210	6	430
Chunky Chicken Salad (¾ cup)	370	27	800
Original Chicken Pot Pie (15 oz)	750	34	2380
Meat Loaf with Brown Gravy (7 oz)	390	22	1040
Ham w/Cinnamon Apples (8 oz)	350	13	1750
Steamed Vegetables (⅔ cup)	40	0	40

	Calories	Fat (g)	Sodium (mg)
BOSTON MARKET *(continued)*			
Herbed Sweet Corn *(¾ cup)*	180	4	170
Rice Pilaf *(⅔ cup)*	180	5	600
Savory Stuffing *(¾ cup)*	310	12	1140
Corn Bread *(1)*	200	6	390
Oatmeal Raisin Cookie *(1)*	320	13	260
Coleslaw *(¾ cup)*	280	16	520
Homestyle Mashed Potatoes *with gravy* *(¾ cup)*	200	9	560
BURGER KING			
BK Broiler	550	29	480
Hamburger	330	15	530
Jr. Whopper *with Cheese*	460	28	770
French Fries *(king size)*	590	30	1110
Whopper	630	39	865
Broiled Chicken Salad with 2 packets Light Italian Dressing	230	11	830
D'ANGELO'S			
Turkey D'Lite Pokket	330	2	490
Turkey D'Lite Small Sub	365	4	535
Roast Beef D'Lite Pokket	330	6	710
Chicken Stir Fry D'Lite Pokket	360	4.5	1240
Classic Vegetable D'Lite Pokket	340	10	960
Turkey D'Lite Super Salad	375	4	660
Tuna D'Lite Super Salad	305	2	805
Chicken D'Lite Super Salad	325	4	980

(Continued)

	Calories	Fat (g)	Sodium (mg)
MCDONALD'S			
Hamburger	270	10	530
Cheeseburger	320	14	730
Chicken McNuggets (9)	430	26	870
Quarter Pounder	420	20	690
Big Mac	530	28	960
Chicken Classic	260	4	500
(no mayonnaise)			
Filet O'Fish	360	16	690
French Fries (small)	210	10	135
Grilled Chicken Salad	170	2	570
(with fat-free Herb			
Vinaigrette)			
Chicken Fajita (1)	190	8	310
SUBWAY			
Veggie Delite 6"	240	3	590
Roast Beef 6"	300	5	940
Club or Ham 6"	310	5	1340
Tuna Sub (with Lite	390	15	940
Mayonnaise) 6"			
Tuna Sub 6"	540	32	890
Turkey Club or Ham	180	4	1230
Salad (with fat-free			
dressing)			
Chicken or Turkey Sub 6"	320	5	1190
PIZZA (2 SLICES OF 12"-DIAMETER PIZZA)			
DOMINO'S			
Cheese	344	10	981
Veggie	373	12	745
LITTLE CAESAR'S			
Pepperoni	220	9	358
Baby Pan	616	24	1466
PIZZA HUT			
Meat Lover's	501	22	1483
Pepperoni Stuffed Crust	460	20	1353

	Calories	**Fat (g)**	**Sodium (mg)**
TACO BELL			
Bean Burrito	390	12	1140
Soft Taco	220	11	540
Mexican Pizza	570	36	1050
Taco Salad *with salsa*	840	52	1670
Steak Fajita Wrap	460	21	1130
WENDY'S			
Grilled Chicken Sandwich	310	8	780
Spicy Chicken Sandwich	410	15	1280
Single Burger *with everything*	420	20	810
Chicken Caesar Pita	490	18	1300
Garden Veggie Pita	400	17	780
Garden Ranch Chicken Pita	480	18	1170
Chili *(small)*	190	6	670
Baked Potato	450	<1	450
Broccoli & Cheese Potato	470	14	470
Chili & Cheese Potato	630	24	770
Bacon & Cheese Potato	530	18	1390
FAMILY STYLE RESTAURANT ITEMS			
Buffalo Wings*(12 wings)*	700	48	1750
Stuffed Potato Skins *(8 skins)*	1120	79	1270
Fried Whole Onion *(3 cups)*	1690	116	3040
Sirloin Steak, trimmed *(12 oz)*	390	15	470
Filet Mignon, trimmed *(9 oz)*	350	18	330
Baked Potato *with* 1 tablespoon sour cream	280	3	200
Caesar Salad *(2 cups)*	310	26	620
Chicken Caesar Salad *(4 cups, with dressing)*	660	46	1490

(Continued)

	Calories	Fat (g)	Sodium (mg)
FAMILY STYLE RESTAURANT ITEMS *(continued)*			
Hamburger *(10 oz)*	660	36	810
Chicken Chow Mein with *Rice (5 cups)*	1005	32	2450
Lasagna *(2 cups)*	960	53	2060

You can use this table (compiled by Mary Card, R.D.) to make better selections the next time you eat at a fast-food restaurant. For example, if you choose the McGrilled Chicken Classic without mayonnaise or oil, it only has 4 grams of fat. A bowl of chili at Wendy's has only 6 grams of fat. If you choose the chili and a baked potato, you have a great lunch with very little fat.

14. Snack Smart

For most people, the evening meal and after-dinner snacking are the things that wreak havoc with both cholesterol and weight. People often tell me that they are so hungry when they get home from work that they grab at the first thing they see. Unfortunately that might be a bag of chips, a handful of cashews, or a few chocolate-chip cookies. This kind of frenzied eating can really add fat to your day.

If you commute to work (or if you are planning to be out all day), I suggest keeping a bottle of water or a diet soda, and a small snack like a piece of fruit, a small bag of pretzels, or a couple of graham crackers, in a cooler for the ride home. Leaving the cooler in the car prevents your eating your snack at three P.M. when you are only a little hungry; you will need it more on the way home. Having a snack in the car will take the edge off your hunger. You will be in a better mood when you get home and will be less likely to grab the first edible thing you see.

15. Dine Out Wisely

Many of my patients eat out several times a week. This can, but need not, be a recipe for disaster. My first advice would be: if you don't have to eat out because of work or travel, limit yourself to once a week. If you are on the road for business or pleasure and have no other option, you *can* dine out without blowing your fat budget, but it takes willpower and a certain degree of assertiveness. You have to be firm with the waitstaff regarding your food preferences.

Look for the following words in the menu: *steamed, stir-fried, barbecued, grilled, broiled,* or *roasted.* While not foolproof, these words are generally used to describe lower-fat choices. It is useful to ask your waitstaff a bit more about the cooking preparation. It should also be obvious that if a very high-fat food is prepared using one of the above methods, it is still going to be high in fat. As an example, barbecued ribs are never a good choice but barbecued skinless chicken may well be.

In contrast to these low-fat cooking methods, the following words or phrases generally describe high-fat cooking methods: *buttery, crispy, fried, in cream sauce, in cheese,* or *stewed.*

Don't be afraid to make special requests. The chef knows that there are many restaurants for you to choose from; the last thing he or she wants is an unhappy customer. About a year ago, my husband and I were taking my parents out for their anniversary. We choose a place called Richard's Bistro—the best "occasion restaurant" in our area and definitely not known for its wide variety of low-fat choices.

I called ahead to ask if Richard might be able to whip up something acceptable for me. The person I spoke to said that would be fine. He asked if a grilled vegetable dish would be something I might like. I thought that sounded great. When it was time to order, the waiter said Richard was aware I was coming and had made something special. What I didn't expect was that Richard would deliver my meal himself, saying, "I just wanted to meet the little lady who doesn't like my cooking." I explained to Richard that it wasn't that I didn't like his cooking; I was sure I was going to enjoy my special dish. I just wanted a lower-fat version of his excellent food. Although I was embarrassed, I stuck to my guns and got what I wanted. If you see something on the menu that would be great without the added gravy, sauce, or dressing, ask for it on the side, and then use only a tiny amount or none at all.

Ask for butter, margarine, mayonnaise, and sour cream to be served on the side too. By eliminating one tablespoon of butter or mayonnaise, you save 100 calories and 14 grams of fat!

Don't be afraid to ask for substitutions. Ask for a baked potato instead of French fries; ask for fruit instead of chips. Request low-fat milk, either as a beverage in its own right or for coffee and tea. Ask for mustard on your sandwich instead of mayonnaise. If a basket of bread or tortilla chips is automatically placed on the table, send it back to the kitchen. If it is there, you will eat it; you are only human, and probably hungry as well!

Limit your portions. There is nothing wrong with two adults splitting a meal. Order a half-portion or a child's portion. One of my patients told me that when dining out on business trips, he always planned to leave half his meal on his plate, but found that once he finished half he continued to pick until—to his surprise—the plate was empty. Now, as soon as his food arrives he asks for a Styrofoam box and places half his meal in it. He does this even if he is staying in a hotel without a refrigerator. He explained to me that this worked for him because he would be too embarrassed to dig into the doggie bag for "just a few more bites." He also told me that it took a lot for him to be bold enough to ask for the Styrofoam box at the start of the meal; I can imagine it was embarrassing. But since he started doing this, he has lost 10 pounds and dropped his LDL cholesterol by 30 mg/dl. A number of his business associates and clients at first thought he was a bit quirky, but now that they see how great he looks they are getting their doggie bags as the main course arrives. Don't be afraid to start a trend. After all, it is your body, your cholesterol, and, most importantly, your arteries that will benefit, so who cares if it is quirky?

16. Make Healthy Choices at Ethnic Restaurants

Whether you are dining out in your own hometown or traveling for business or pleasure, ethnic foods can be adventurous and fun. They can introduce you to a variety of new food choices. Sometimes the food names or descriptions can be a little confusing. Don't hesitate to ask the waiter what a food is or how it is prepared.

Here are a few tips for dining in Italian, Chinese, Mexican, and Indian restaurants.

Italian

Begin by sending back the bread and ordering a salad. Good choices include an arugula and Belgian endive salad, or the house salad. (Ask for the dressing on the side.) An *insalata frutte di mare* (seafood in a light marinade served on greens) is another low-fat choice. Many Italian soups are low in fat. Try minestrone, *pasta e fagioli*, or tortellini in broth. Eat slowly, enjoy your dining companions, and don't be afraid to leave food in your bowl or on your plate.

As you move on to the main course, remember shrimp is your friend. Try shrimp primavera or shrimp in marinara sauce. Sole primavera is generally another excellent low-fat entrée. Consider ordering pasta with marinara sauce (no meat or cheese). Other excellent choices include linguine with white clam sauce, chicken in wine sauce, and chicken or veal cacciatore. Instead of spumoni or anything with cream in it, end with a sorbet or Italian ice.

Chinese

Chinese food can seem deceptively healthy. It's traditionally very healthy, and obesity is relatively rare in Chinese populations. That's because most Chinese people living in China get lots of exercise, eat mainly rice and vegetables, and don't go out to eat at Chinese restaurants in America. However, you *can* easily make good, low-fat choices at a Chinese restaurant. The trick is to focus on what the thin Chinese eat themselves: vegetables, rice, and noodles. When it comes to rice and noodles, though, remember that even though they are low in fat they do have calories. Watch the portion size, and ask for brown rice if available.

Begin with the steamed Peking ravioli. Soup is also an excellent way to start your meal in a Chinese restaurant. A few good choices are hot and sour soup, wonton, sizzling rice, and delights of three. For your main course, stay away from entrées made using red meat. Instead, order teriyaki or Yu-Hsiang chicken. Chicken or vegetable lo mein is generally also a lower-fat entrée. Shrimp is frequently featured on the menu in Chinese restaurants. Go with the shrimp with broccoli, moo shoo shrimp, or Szechwan shrimp. Vegetable stir-fries, with or without tofu, can also be an excellent selection.

Mexican

Mexican food is notoriously high in fat. Nevertheless, it is possible to get in and out of most Mexican restaurants without blowing your fat budget. (Women should aim to limit it to no more than 27 grams per day, and most men should set 35 grams as the limit. Growing children are typically allowed 40 grams per day.)

Rule number one in a Mexican restaurant: send back the chips. It is amazing how you can find the basket of tortilla chips empty even when you only planned to eat one or two. It has happened to all of us. Rule number two: if it is covered with cheese, it has a million grams of fat (that's a little bit of an exaggeration, but only a little). Don't order it. Keep your order simple and as devoid of melted cheese as possible. Instead of starting with the chips, begin with gazpacho, black-bean soup, chili, or a dinner salad with the dressing on the side. Go with Mexican rice. Eat as much salsa as you want. Ask for flour or corn tortillas. In general, the chicken fajitas, enchiladas, and burritos are fine as long as you make sure to limit the cheese.

It is not just the cheese that will kill you in a Mexican restaurant; make sure you hold the sour cream, guacamole, and refried beans. Many Mexican restaurants are now offering low-fat sour cream and low-fat or fat-free refried beans.

Don't be afraid to ask. In most cases you won't be able to tell the difference between the high-fat and low-fat versions of these products.

Indian

North Indian food is generally much richer than that of the South. In the North they tend to use a great deal of *ghee* (clarified butter). Northern Indians also prefer flaky and fried breads (*puris* and *parathas*). Southern Indian cuisine tends to favor rice instead of bread. *Chappatties*, however, can be found all over the country and are virtually fat-free.

Indian restaurants in America are usually either North Indian or South Indian; you seldom find both cuisines in one place. But Indian chefs are accustomed to dealing with many special requests. (Jains, for example, eat no garlic or onions — staple items in restaurant food — but this doesn't stop them from eating out.) So don't be afraid to ask for what you want. In addition to the low-fat breads just mentioned, try the *raitas* (chopped vegetable salads in spiced yogurt).They are an especially good choice if they are made with low-fat yogurt. Avoid *boondi ki raita*. Ask for your lentils (*dal*) to be served without the *tarka* (spices fried in oil and added at the last minute). Ask which vegetables are served *suki* (without gravy), and order those. *Idli*, a steamed rice and lentil cake, is a part of a delicious nonfat meal served with lentil soup and chutneys. Chutneys are typically fat-free (except for the coconut ones), but can be very spicy.

17. Eat More Walnuts

In 1992 Dr. G. E. Fraser, J. Sabaté, and colleagues from the Center for Health Research at the University of California's School of Public Health found that Seventh-Day Adventists (vegetarians because of their religious convictions) who consumed nuts on a regular basis had a markedly lower risk of developing a cardiac event than people in the general population.

One year later the same group compared the impact of a low-fat, walnut-rich diet to a low-fat diet without nuts in a group of healthy young men. The study appeared in the *New England Journal of Medicine* in March 1993. It showed that a low-fat diet containing walnuts as the main fat source (55 percent of fat calories came from walnuts) resulted in a 22.4 mg/dl reduction in total cholesterol as compared to the standard low-fat diet.

Because these first two studies contained very specific groups of individuals (Seventh-Day Adventists and young males), some in the scientific community questioned whether these findings might be applicable to the general population. In order to address this issue, Drs. Zambon and Sabaté designed an elegant trial that included middle-aged men and women with elevated cholesterol. Forty-nine people participated in the trial, which examined the impact of three different diets.

Participants were initially asked to follow either a low-fat Mediterranean diet or a low-fat diet in which walnuts represented 55 percent of fat calories. (Depending on a person's calorie allowance, this meant consuming between eight and eleven walnuts per day.)

After six weeks, participants were switched to the alternate diet. As you might imagine, the Mediterranean diet had a heavy emphasis on fish and vegetables. Olive oil was a major fat source. Red meat and eggs were used in very limited amounts, and nuts were not allowed. Table 5 shows the results of this study:

**TABLE 5 Comparison of the Effects of
Mediterranean and Walnut Diets
on Cholesterol**

Cholesterol Levels	Baseline	Mediterranean Diet	Walnut Diet
Total cholesterol	279 ± 32	264 ± 31	253 ± 35
Triglycerides	134 ± 38	134 ± 44	126 ± 44
LDL cholesterol	195 ± 29	185 ± 25	174 ± 30
HDL cholesterol	56 ± 12	53 ± 12	55 ± 14

Adapted with permission from a study by D. Zambon, J. Sabaté, and S. Munoz: "Substituting walnuts for monounsaturated fat improves the serum lipid profile of hypercholesterolemic men and women." *Annals of Internal Medicine* 132, 2000: 538–546.

It is impossible for me to say that you will have exactly a 26 mg/dl drop in your total cholesterol and a 21 mg/dl drop in your LDL cholesterol if you add walnuts to your diet; however, the evidence looks quite convincing. Keep in mind that the walnuts must replace other fats already in your diet. If you simply add the walnuts without getting rid of some other fat source, you are likely to simply gain weight and may even increase your cholesterol level. In order to incorporate walnuts into your diet, you really have to love them because on a 20-percent-fat diet there is not much room for other fat sources.

If you want to try the walnut experiment, I recommend that you add eight walnuts per day and remove 20 grams of fat and 200 calories from your current diet. (Each walnut contains 25 calories and 2.5 grams of fat.) After about six weeks, you will be able to see the impact of your dietary change. Ask your doctor to order a full-fasting cholesterol profile.

In addition to their cholesterol-lowering potential, walnuts have another potential mechanism for providing you with cardiovascular protection. No other nut contains as much alpha-linolenic acid. Alpha-linolenic acid appears to be able to prevent platelets from clumping together. Platelets are our blood-clotting cells, so preventing them from clumping together might prevent a blood clot from forming. Most heart attacks occur when a cholesterol plaque cracks open and a blood clot forms on top, leading to a complete blockage in a person's heart artery. By preventing the platelets from clumping together, one important part of the heart attack equation might be reversed.

Walnuts, then, appear to favorably alter risk in two ways. First, they lower the cholesterol level; second, they may prevent blood clots from occurring.

18. Get More Soy Protein in Your Diet

The cholesterol-lowering effects of soy protein have been recognized for a long time. Studies conducted by Sirtori and colleagues and by Verrillo and colleagues found that people with high cholesterol might lower their total cholesterol by as much as 23 to 30 percent if most or all of their protein intake was replaced by soy protein.

In a country like the United States, where most people get little or none of their protein from soy, people are unlikely to be willing to replace all of their dietary protein with soy sources. So it was an important discovery when a study done in 1993 by Dr. Susan Potter at the University of Illinois found that partial replacement of animal protein with soy protein resulted in a 12 percent reduction in cholesterol.

None of the aforementioned studies were large; they ranged from 19 to 65 participants. In order to determine if soy protein could truly be expected to reduce cholesterol significantly, James Anderson, M.D., conducted a meta-analysis of 38 studies, including the small studies mentioned on the previous page. A meta-analysis is a complex but very useful way to answer questions in medicine. Although it's not a perfect method, a meta-analysis can be used to try to answer a question if only small studies have been performed.

In the case of soy protein, none of the 38 studies Dr. Anderson examined was big enough to definitively answer the soy/cholesterol question on its own; however, when pooled together, an answer emerged. To be included in the meta-analysis, a study had to have been rigorously conducted. The studies Dr. Anderson looked at contained between 4 and 127 participants each, with 740 participants in all. Each consumed between 17 and 124 grams of soy per day; the average was 47 grams.

Dr. Anderson's meta-analysis, which was published in the prestigious *New England Journal of Medicine* in August 1995, found that the replacement of animal protein with soy protein resulted in a significant reduction in total cholesterol levels (9.3 percent) and LDL cholesterol (12.9 percent). Triglyceride levels also fell significantly (10.5 percent). The higher a person's initial cholesterol readings, the greater the impact of soy protein. In fact, in the people with the highest cholesterol levels (above 335 mg/dl), as much as a 24 percent reduction in LDL cholesterol was seen.

Dr. Anderson's meta-analysis prompted the Food and Drug Administration (FDA) to look more closely at soy foods. In 1998 the FDA determined that soy protein, as part of a diet low in saturated fat and cholesterol, is likely to reduce blood cholesterol levels and consequently to reduce the risk of coronary heart disease. Based on this determination, the FDA began allowing soy-food manufacturers to print health claims on their products. After determining that 25 grams per day of soy protein was enough to promote cholesterol reduction, the FDA proposed the following template for health claims. "Twenty-five grams of soy protein a day, as part of a diet low in saturated fat and cholesterol, may reduce the risk of heart disease. A serving of (name of food) supplies _____ grams of soy protein." An alternative would read something like this: "Diets low in saturated fat and cholesterol that include 25 grams of soy protein per day may reduce the risk of heart disease. One serving of (name of food) provides _____ grams of soy protein." The FDA now recommends that four servings of at least 6.25 grams each of soy protein be added to a diet low in saturated fat and cholesterol.

Since the FDA's initial recommendation in 1998, many scientists have tried to determine the mechanism by which soy protein lowers cholesterol. More research is needed, but it now appears that the isoflavone content of soy protein is the key to cholesterol reduction. (Isoflavones are naturally occurring hormone-like substances.)

Dr. John Crouse III presented his important findings regarding the role of isoflavones at the American Heart Association's 38th annual conference on Cardiovascular Disease, Epidemiology, and Prevention, held in Santa Fe, New Mexico. Dr. Crouse and colleagues presented a study of 156 men and women whose total and LDL cholesterol levels hovered around 241 mg/dl and 164 mg/dl, respectively. Participants were randomly assigned to drink one of five liquids per day for a total of nine weeks. Each liquid contained 25 grams of protein. Group One drank a liquid containing 25 grams of protein from cow's milk. Groups

Two through Five drank a liquid containing soy protein. The only difference between the soy-protein groups' liquids was the amount of isoflavones contained in the liquid. The isoflavone content ranged from 4 to 62 mg; (Group Two = 4 mg, Group Three = 27 mg, Group Four = 37 mg, and Group Five = 62 mg.) Dr. Crouse and colleagues found that neither the milk protein group nor the group whose soy protein contained only 4 mg of isoflavones had any reduction in cholesterol. Groups Three, Four, and Five all experienced significant reduction in cholesterol — and the greater the isoflavone content of the liquid, the greater the reduction in cholesterol.

The isoflavones may be essential for soy protein to exert its cholesterol-lowering effect, but this should not be taken to mean that all that is needed to lower cholesterol is the isoflavones. Much more research is needed to determine exactly how soy foods exert their cholesterol-lowering impact. Until that time, I feel the best advice I can give my patients is to incorporate whole soy foods (which contain isoflavones rather than isoflavone supplements) into their diets.

The average person in America consumes between one and three grams of soy protein per day. This is in sharp contrast to East Asia, where soy has been a part of the typical Asian diet for more than four thousand years. In Japan, it is common for people to consume up to 50 grams of soy per day. Because it is unlikely that you plan to move to Japan, it is logical for you to ask, "How can I incorporate soy into my American diet?" This is exactly the question my patients usually ask.

I find that the easiest way for most people to incorporate soy foods into their diet is by making substitutions. I first encourage people to experiment with soymilk. (I recommend the low-fat varieties.) Soymilk tastes quite different from cow's milk, so it may take a little time for you to enjoy it. People frequently need to try a few different brands of soymilk before they find one they really like. Be patient; your palate can grow to love soymilk. One great way to add soymilk to your diet is to add fruit and ice and blend the mixture into a fruit smoothie. An eight-ounce glass of soymilk contains between six and eight grams of soy protein.

Soy burgers, breakfast sausages, and hot dogs are another great choice. Again, there are many varieties of both the burgers and the hot dogs. Each burger, sausage, or hot dog provides between six and ten grams of soy protein per serving. Add one of these and you are more than halfway to your goal.

In addition to the burgers, soy crumbles (pieces of soy burgers crumbled up and ready to add to pasta sauce) are also available. For people who find it hard to give up their meat sauce, I recommend mixing low-fat red meat with the crumbles. Your family is unlikely to notice the healthy change.

Soy nuts are also delicious. I pop them in my children's lunch almost every day. One-fourth of a cup of soy nuts provides 12 grams of soy protein. (You could add half a cup and be at your goal, but because soy nuts have quite a lot of calories you might be better off with one-eighth of a cup.)

Soy cheeses and yogurts are also great and are available in many different flavors. A serving of soy cheese or yogurt typically contains five to six grams of soy protein.

Another great-tasting soy product is soy-nut butter. This is an excellent alternative to peanut butter. Two tablespoons of soy-nut butter contain about eight grams of soy protein.

Soy flour can easily be used in baking; one-fourth of a cup contains about seven grams of soy protein. For people who are interested in trying new foods, I recommend tofu. Four ounces contain between eight and eleven grams of soy protein. Another good choice is tempeh, which contains a whopping 16 grams of soy protein. Tempeh, an Indonesian food, is a rich, flat cake made from fermented soybeans that are typically mixed with rice, millet, or barley. The mixture has a distinctive nutty flavor. I frequently enjoy tempeh in a stir-fry, where it easily replaces chicken.

If you are interested in more information on incorporating soy into your diet, including lots of recipes, there is a wealth of information available online. I recommend the following websites:

talksoy.com (United Soybean Board)

soyohio.org (Ohio Soybean Council)

soyfoods.com (Indiana Soybean Board)

ilsoy.org (Illinois Soybean Association)

michigansoybean.org (Michigan Soybean Association)

If you are not connected to the Internet, call 1-800-TALK-SOY (1-800-825-5769) for information.

19. Increase Your Fiber Intake

Dietary fiber received a great deal of media attention a few years ago. You probably remember the oat-bran craze. Fiber is a lot more than just oat bran, however. Fiber is a rather nondescript term used to categorize a group of carbohydrates that are not digestible by the human digestive system. You are probably aware that certain types of fiber have been reported to lower cholesterol. But how does fiber lower cholesterol? What fiber source is best? And how much should you be eating to achieve a meaningful cholesterol reduction?

Although there is no doubt that dietary fiber will lower cholesterol, its precise mechanism of action is not totally understood. It does appear that fiber can bind bile acids. Bile acids are made in the liver from cholesterol. Each time we eat, bile acids are shipped to the gallbladder and into the intestines, where they help digest the food. Normally, after we digest our food, we reabsorb the bile acids and use them over again. Fiber seems to bind the bile acids, which means that instead of being reabsorbed they are passed out in the stool. The liver must then recruit cholesterol from the bloodstream to make more bile acids. This ultimately results in a reduction in the blood cholesterol level.

Another line of evidence suggests that the fiber is fermented in the intestines by bacteria that naturally live there. This process may produce fatty acids, which in turn seem to prevent the liver from producing cholesterol.

Finally, although it's clearly only part of the story, fiber creates a sense of fullness that may allow a person to eat a little less and may also replace fat in the diet. This might result in weight loss, which would lower cholesterol, and in a lower fat intake, which would again lower cholesterol.

Dietary fiber comes in two types: water-soluble and water-insoluble. Water-soluble fiber has been shown to lower cholesterol, whereas water-insoluble fiber has not. Good sources of water-soluble fiber include legumes (pinto, white, kidney, garbanzo, and other beans, as well as peas), rolled oats, oat bran, pectin (found in fruits such as apples, grapefruit, and oranges), and gums. (Guar gum is the most common. It comes from the guar seed and is commonly used as a food thickener in the United States.) Psyllium, which is derived from the husks of certain seeds, is another important source of water-soluble fiber. It is unlikely that you consume psyllium as part of the food in your diet, but if you have ever taken a bulk laxative such as Metamucil, you have taken psyllium. Psyllium is the main ingredient of Metamucil and is sometimes added to cereals to increase their fiber content.

The most common source of water-insoluble fiber in the American diet is wheat bran. This type of fiber may be useful in preventing constipation, but it will not lower cholesterol.

In reality, most high-fiber foods contain both soluble and insoluble fibers. In general, if you consume 25 grams of fiber per day (as long it isn't all in the form of wheat bran), you will experience a meaningful (5 to 15 percent) reduction in your cholesterol level. The degree of reduction depends in part on how well you respond to fiber (not everyone has the same response) and on how much fiber you already have in your baseline diet.

If you are like most Americans, your current fiber intake is quite low, typically on the order of 10 to 12 grams per day. If this is your situation, you are very likely to improve your cholesterol level as you increase to 25 grams of fiber per day. As you add fiber to your diet, it is essential that you take it slowly. If you dramatically increase your fiber intake overnight, you are likely to experience abdominal fullness, bloating, and gas. These unpleasant feelings are minimized if you gradually increase your fiber intake over the course of a month or so. It is also important for you to drink lots of water as you increase your intake of water-soluble fiber. The fiber acts like a sponge to soak up water. This characteristic creates the full feeling (making you less hungry) and helps the fiber perform its cholesterol-lowering job.

Because there are so many different types of water-soluble fiber, you may wonder if one type is better at lowering cholesterol than another. This is not an easy question to answer. As I prepared this book, I reviewed more than one hundred studies that utilized many different types of water-soluble fiber. No two studies were exactly alike. The studies examined different types of fiber, different doses of fiber, different populations of people (old, young, with high cholesterol, with normal cholesterol levels, men, women). With all these variables, it is almost impossible to predict in any given person what kind of a response a particular dose of water-soluble fiber will produce. For example, Dr. James Anderson from the University of Kentucky, probably the world's authority on fiber, has reported as much as a 20 percent reduction in LDL cholesterol in test subjects after they consumed 10.2 grams of psyllium per day for eight weeks. This study was performed in men with high cholesterol. Other investigators testing the same dose, or higher doses, of psyllium in different populations have found reductions in LDL cholesterol of between 9 and 20 percent.

In a series of clinical trials in differing patient populations, Dr. Anderson found that navy and pinto beans (dose range from 50 to 115 grams per day) could lower the LDL cholesterol by between 13 and 24 percent.

And in studies lasting up to two years, large quantities of oat bran have been found to lower LDL cholesterol by as much as 29 percent.

Because it is so difficult to compare fiber studies, I suggest the following. Consume a wide variety of high-fiber foods daily. As mentioned earlier, aim for at least 25 grams of fiber per day. (More fiber is even better). Table 6 will be helpful as you choose your favorite high-fiber foods:

TABLE 6 Fiber Content of Foods

Food	Amount	Soluble Fiber (g)	Total Fiber (g)
LEGUMES (COOKED)			
Kidney beans	½ cup	2.8	6.9
Lima beans	½ cup	2.7	6.9
Black beans	½ cup	2.4	6.1
Navy beans	½ cup	2.2	6.5
Pinto beans	½ cup	1.9	5.9
Chickpeas	½ cup	1.3	4.3
CEREALS AND GRAINS			
Oatmeal (dry)	⅓ cup	1.3	2.8
Cheerios	1 cup	1.0	2.0
Oat bran (dry)	⅓ cup	2.0	4.4
Brown rice (cooked)	½ cup	0.4	5.3
Whole-wheat bread	1 slice	0.4	2.1
White bread	1 slice	0.2	0.4
FRUIT			
Apple	1 medium	1.2	3.6
Orange	1 medium	1.8	2.9
Grapefruit	1 medium	2.2	3.6
Grapes	1 cup	0.3	1.1
Prunes	6 medium	3.0	8.0
Banana	1 medium	0.6	1.9
Raisins	¼ cup	1.0	2.0
VEGETABLES (COOKED)			
Brussels sprouts	½ cup	2.0	3.8
Broccoli	½ cup	1.1	2.6
Carrots	½ cup	1.5	3.2
Spinach	½ cup	0.5	2.1
Sweet potato	1 medium	1.1	2.5
Zucchini	½ cup	0.2	1.6

Food	Amount	Soluble Fiber (g)	Total Fiber (g)
FIBER SUPPLEMENTS			
Sugar Free Metamucil	1 tablespoon	5.2	6.0
Citrus Pectin	1 tablespoon	5.5	5.5
Profibre	1 scoop	5.0	5.0
Citrucel	1 tablespoon	2.0	2.0

Finally, note that foods that are rich in fiber contain more than just fiber. Many contain compounds called saponins. Saponins are compounds that occur in plants and have the ability to bind cholesterol in the intestine, thereby preventing absorption.

20. Be Cautious with Alcohol

Many people are in the habit of having an alcoholic beverage before dinner, in the spirit of heart health. By now most people have heard that alcohol is good for the heart. It is true that there is some relatively strong evidence supporting the notion that alcohol consumption may reduce cardiac risk. While the mechanisms by which alcohol protects against cardiovascular events are not totally worked out, it appears that alcohol's ability to raise blood levels of both HDL cholesterol (the good cholesterol) and tissue plasminogen activator (TPA) are important. TPA is a natural clot-dissolver. Most heart attacks are caused by the combination of a cholesterol deposit and a blood clot on top (the result being a completely blocked artery), so having high blood levels of TPA would clearly be beneficial. Alcohol also seems to prevent platelets, the blood's clotting cells, from clumping together.

But although alcohol probably does provide some cardiovascular protection, it is equally important to look at the negative aspects of alcohol as you decide whether a drink a day is a good philosophy for you. Alcohol tends to raise blood levels of sugar and triglycerides. Alcohol can cause blood pressure to rise and has been linked to breast cancer in women. Heavy alcohol consumption can increase the risk of cardiomyopathy (an unhealthy enlargement of the heart), heart arrhythmias (electrical disturbances within the heart), cirrhosis of the liver, pancreatitis, gastritis, some forms of stroke, and cancer of the mouth, pharynx, larynx, esophagus, and liver.

If you decide you are going to have a nightly alcoholic beverage, I would suggest that you have it after dinner rather than before dinner. Because alcohol is an appetite stimulant, drinking it on an empty stomach may mean you consume more calories than you care to at dinner. And don't forget that alcohol has calories too (see Table 7):

TABLE 7 Caloric Content of Alcohol

6 oz wine (white):	approximately 150 calories
6 oz wine (red):	approximately 150 calories
12 oz beer:	approximately 150 calories
12 oz beer (light):	approximately 100 calories
1.5 oz hard liquor (80 proof):	approximately 100 calories
1.5 oz hard liquor (90 proof):	approximately 110 calories

PART THREE

Supplements

21. Consider Supplements

Sometimes no matter how hard a person tries, his or her cholesterol level remains stubbornly high. Many people ask me if dietary supplements would play a role in reducing their cholesterol. The answer is "yes." Dietary or herbal supplements are more aptly termed "nutraceuticals." With roughly 20 percent of adults in the United States taking an estimated four billion dollars' worth of these nutraceuticals, the supplement market is truly big business. It is crucial for you to know how these supplements work and how well they work.

Most nutraceuticals have only a modest impact on a person's cholesterol profile. However, patients can frequently avoid medications if several different nutraceuticals are used in conjunction with a low-fat and (when necessary) low-sugar diet and a sensible exercise program. The important point to remember is that just as a diet only works when a person is faithful to it, nutraceuticals or supplements will only work when taken properly and consistently.

22. Talk to Your Doctor About Cholestin

To be honest, I am not sure if Cholestin really belongs here in the supplements section, even though it *is* an over-the-counter product. In my opinion, Cholestin is really a drug; as such, if you choose to take Cholestin, your doctor should know you are doing so. He or she will want to periodically check your cholesterol profile and liver functions.

Cholestin is a red yeast (*Monascus purpureus*) fermented on rice. This is the "spice" that gives Peking duck its distinctive red color. It is also a key ingredient in Chinese rice wine. Red yeast fermented on rice has been used for centuries in China, both in cooking and as a medicine. Interestingly, one of the key ingredients of Cholestin is mevinolin, a compound almost identical to lovastatin (Mevacor). Mevacor, as you might know, is a powerful cholesterol-lowering medication in the family of drugs known as *statins*. (See introduction.) Other drugs in this family include atorvastatin (Lipitor), simvastatin (Zocor), fluvastatin (Lescol) and pravastatin (Pravachol). All of them are discussed in Part Six of this book.

Cholestin came on the market in 1997 with a big media splash. Pharmanex, Inc., the manufacturer of Cholestin, took out large ads in many popular magazines. The media blitz caught the attention of the Food and Drug Administration (FDA). Given Cholestin's claim to reduce cholesterol levels by 25 to 40 points, and its chemical similarity to the cholesterol-lowering *drug* Mevacor, the FDA became involved, deciding that Cholestin was a drug and should be regulated as such. As the FDA prepared to have Cholestin taken off the shelves of drug stores and health-food stores, Pharmanex, Inc., challenged the FDA in court. To many people's surprise, in February of 1999, a federal judge in Salt Lake City, Utah, ruled in favor of Pharmanex. (Pharmanex has since been purchased by Nu Skin International of Provo, Utah.)

At this point you probably have little doubt that Cholestin works (given its similarity to Mevacor). But you may be wondering *how* it works. You may also wonder how well it works, and if it has side effects. Just like Mevacor, Cholestin works by blocking a key enzyme involved in cholesterol biosynthesis (production) in the liver. This enzyme is called HMG CoA Reductase. Both Mevacor and Cholestin partially block this enzyme; the end result is that less cholesterol is produced in your liver.

Cholestin, Mevacor, and all the drugs in the statin family also increase the number of LDL receptors on the liver cells. The LDL receptors remove LDL cholesterol (the bad cholesterol) from the bloodstream. As you increase the dose of any statin medication, you lower blood cholesterol levels more effectively.

Cholestin, when taken as directed by the manufacturer (two 600-mg capsules twice a day for a total of 2,400 mg per day), will lower the LDL cholesterol by 21 percent. This is roughly equivalent to low-dose Mevacor.

When Cholestin first came out in 1997, all the studies cited came from China. Because people in China typically have a very different diet than people in the United States, it is crucial to know if Cholestin works as well in the United States as it does in China. The answer is that it appears to work equally well.

In February of 1999, Dr. David Heber of the University of California published a report in the *American Journal of Clinical Nutrition.* His study involved 83 volunteers. After eight weeks on Cholestin, participants averaged a 17 percent reduction in their total cholesterol level.

In March of 1999, a second U.S. study was presented at an American Heart Association meeting in Orlando, Florida. Dr. James Rippe, a cardiologist at Tufts University School of Medicine in Boston, conducted the study. It included 233 people (treated at 12 different medical centers) whose average baseline cholesterol was 242 mg/dl and whose baseline LDL cholesterol level was 158 mg/dl. After eight weeks on Cholestin, the subjects' average total cholesterol had fallen by 16.4 percent to 206 mg/dl. The average LDL cholesterol fell an impressive 21 percent to 125 mg/dl. The HDL cholesterol level of participants was also positively affected, increasing by 14.6 percent during the eight-week study. Baseline HDL cholesterol was 50 mg/dl; at the conclusion of the study it was 57 mg/dl.

One of my favorite patients is George, a 73-year-old retired accountant who keeps close track of his cholesterol levels. George was very resistant to the idea of taking any cholesterol-lowering medications. The first time I met him, his cholesterol profile looked like this:

George's Level	Desirable Level
Total cholesterol 255 mg/dl	< 200 mg/dl
Triglycerides 160 mg/dl	< 150 mg/dl
LDL cholesterol 189 mg/dl	< 130 mg/dl
HDL cholesterol 34 mg/dl	> 45 mg/dl

George worked extremely hard to improve both his diet and exercise program. He limited his fat to no more than 30 grams per day (often consuming less), and he developed a daily walking program (generally walking an hour a day). The best he was able to achieve with his excellent lifestyle program was:

George's Level	Desirable Level
Total cholesterol 213 mg/dl	< 200 mg/dl
Triglycerides 108 mg/dl	< 150 mg/dl
LDL cholesterol 153 mg/dl	< 130 mg/dl
HDL cholesterol 38 mg/dl	> 45 mg/dl

These levels were clearly better, but they did not satisfy either George (remember, he is an accountant) or me. George asked me what I thought of Cholestin. I told him I thought it was a good product and mentioned the recent studies. I told him that I felt it was reasonable for him to try Cholestin, and suggested that we see each other three months later to check his cholesterol levels and his liver functions. This is his follow-up lipid profile:

George's Level	Desirable Level
Total cholesterol 184 mg/dl	< 200 mg/dl
Triglycerides 86 mg/dl	< 150 mg/dl
LDL cholesterol 121 mg/dl	< 130 mg/dl
HDL cholesterol 45 mg/dl	> 45 mg/dl

It is only fair to say that George intensified his exercise program at the same time that he began the Cholestin, but I am sure the Cholestin improved his HDL cholesterol.

Just as the statin drugs are in general very safe, Cholestin appears to be relatively unlikely to cause serious side effects. (See page xx in the Introduction.) However, you should be aware that drugs in the statin family can cause liver toxicity, although rarely. Even more rare is the occurrence of muscle inflammation (myositis) or muscle destruction (rhabdomyolysis). For the most part, the liver toxicity and myositis are totally reversible if caught early. Rhabdomyolysis, however, can be deadly.

In both of its U.S. trials, Cholestin was remarkably well-tolerated and relatively free from side effects. The major reported side effects were mild gastrointestinal complaints such as gas, cramping, and bloating. A few people complained of mild headache. Neither trial reported any occurrences of significant liver or muscle difficulties.

The bottom line is that although Cholestin is still available to consumers without a prescription, it should probably be thought of as a drug. The current owner of Cholestin, Nu Skin International, has actually removed Cholestin from chain drugstores. Cholestin is currently available only through mail-order and in some independent pharmacies. You can call 1-800-800-0191 for information on Cholestin.

If you decide Cholestin is for you, please:

1. Tell your doctor.

2. Don't take another drug in the statin family at the same time.

3. Ask to have your liver functions tested (a simple blood test) three months after beginning Cholestin and at least twice a year thereafter.

4. Follow a low-fat diet.

5. Stick to the recommended dose of 2,400 mg per day (two 600-mg capsules twice a day).

If you think you are experiencing a side effect related to the Cholestin, stop the drug and contact your doctor.

23. Substitute Benecol and Take Control for Butter and Margarine

Two of the most powerful true nutraceuticals are plant stanols and plant sterols (currently available in Benecol Light and Take Control margarines). Plant stanols and sterols are products derived from vegetable oils and wood pulp. They lower LDL cholesterol by inhibiting cholesterol absorption from the intestine.

The plant stanols and sterols have been studied for about forty years. In the 1950s, early human studies were undertaken. The problem was that scientists felt large quantities of the sterols had to be ingested. The early studies often used up to 18 grams of the plant sterols per day, a quantity far greater than the two to three grams per day suggested now. These early studies proved that plant sterols could lower cholesterol; however, the large doses that were felt necessary at that time were taken as powders, liquid suspensions, and granules, which made them fairly unappealing.

In 1977 Drs. Ann and Bob Lees published their very important research findings in the prestigious journal *Atherosclerosis*. The Lees found that much lower doses (as few as three grams) were just as effective as the much higher doses previously used.

Unfortunately, not much more research on plant stanols and sterols was done until the mid-1980s and early 1990s. The probable reason that these substances were not more aggressively pursued as cholesterol-lowering agents is that people simply did not enjoy taking the powders, liquid suspensions, and granules. This all changed when Mattson and colleagues proposed that the best way to deliver plant stanols/sterols was via dietary fat. In the early 1990s, a group of Finnish investigators developed two products containing plant stanols—a mayonnaise and a margarine. Almost simultaneously, the Lipton Company developed plant sterol margarine. Ultimately, the margarine products were the bigger hit.

Plant stanols and plant sterols are structurally almost identical to cholesterol. They actually compete with cholesterol to form *mixed micelles*. (In order for cholesterol to be absorbed back into the bloodstream from your intestines, it must be packaged in something called a mixed micelle. If your dietary cholesterol doesn't find its way into a micelle, it will simply pass out in your stool.) Plant stanols and sterols do an excellent job preventing the absorption of dietary cholesterol. They are, however, very poorly absorbed themselves. As a result, after they do their job, most of the stanols or sterols you ingest will pass out of your body in your stool.

We eat plant stanols and sterols every day. They are natural substances found in wood, vegetables, vegetable oils, rice, beans, corn, and other plants. In order to significantly lower cholesterol, however, they must be consumed in quantities higher than our typical daily intake. Most people in the United States consume between 160 and 360 mg of plant sterols every day.

Vegetarian cultures that rely heavily on corn and beans consume much higher quantities of plant sterols. For example, the Tarahumara Indians consume as much as 500 mg of plant sterols per day, largely through corn and beans. In order to achieve a meaningful reduction in cholesterol (about a 10 to 14 percent reduction in LDL), we ask people to consume between two and three grams of plant sterols or stanols per day. This is the equivalent of two to three tablespoons of plant stanol or sterol margarines.

As mentioned, the margarines go by the trade names of Benecol (a plant stanol margarine) and Take Control (a plant sterol margarine). When I ask people to begin using these margarines, I get one of two reactions. If we have just met the person, he or she often says, "I really don't want to give up my butter." This tends to be an easy sell. I ask them to just make the substitution until our next visit. The margarines both taste good, so by the time the person returns for a second visit and sees the progress that's been made, he or she doesn't mind continuing with the margarine.

On the other hand, I have many patients whom I have been seeing for years. Many of these people have completely given up margarine or are using only scant amounts of the "I Can't Believe It's Not Butter Light" spray. Asking these people to add back a product that has both fat and calories makes them worry about my sanity. For these people, I point out that there are light versions of both Benecol and Take Control. Two tablespoons of Benecol Light will add about 10 grams of fat and about 90 calories to a person's day. Regular Benecol runs about 18 grams of fat for two tablespoons, so the light version is preferable. The same quantity of Take Control Light will add about nine grams of fat and 80 calories. For most people, this amount of calories can be worked into the diet without fear of weight gain. I explain that even *with* the added fat, their LDL cholesterol will fall. If you compare the two margarines, Benecol has a slight edge in terms of the percentage reduction in LDL. Benecol tends to lower LDL by about 14 percent, while Take Control lowers it by about 10 percent.

Supplements only work if taken religiously. Sometimes people fail to see an improvement with Benecol or Take Control. In almost all cases, the reason is that they are not using enough of the margarine. In order to see an effect, you must use two to three tablespoons per day — every day.

24. Try Basikol or Other Phytosterols

For those of you who travel extensively and cannot bring Benecol or Take Control with you, or if you simply cannot imagine using two to three tablespoons of margarine a day, consider using other forms of phytosterols (plant sterols).

One such phytosterol is Basikol. Basikol has the potential to lower LDL cholesterol as much as Benecol. It is available as a vanilla-flavored powder, which can be sprinkled on cereal or other food, stirred into yogurt, or taken by the scoop with a meal. The good thing about Basikol is that each scoop has only five calories, but contains 800 mg of phytosterols. I recommend between two and three scoops per day with food. This amount should help you achieve a 10 to 14 percent reduction in your LDL cholesterol.

Basikol is distributed by Health from the Sun, a division of the French company Arkopharma. A one-month supply of Basikol (if you are taking two scoops a day) will cost $29.99. It can be ordered by calling (888) 655-2756 or online at healthfromthesun.com. If you prefer to take a capsule instead of the powder, you will be happy to know that a capsule form of Basikol will soon be available.

Other pill or capsule forms of plant sterols include Kholesterol Blocker (each tablet contains 400 mg of plant sterols), available at cholesterol.homepage.com; Source Naturals Phytosterol Complex (each tablet contains 625 mg of plant sterols), available at mothernature.com; and Natrol BetaSitosterol (each tablet contains 415 mg of plant sterols), available at vitaminshoppe.com.

If you are going to use plant stanols or sterols, it is crucial for you to think of them as a prescription and use them as directed.

25. Try Flaxseed

Whole or ground flaxseed appears to have potential as a nutraceutical. As opposed to flaxseed oil, which has been shown to have only very modest cholesterol-lowering potential, whole and ground flaxseed has been shown in a few small studies to lower LDL cholesterol by almost 15 percent, when incorporated into the diet in baked goods or sprinkled on cereal, yogurt, or vegetables.

Although all the mechanisms by which flaxseed leads to a reduction in cholesterol have not been fully worked out, some things are known. Flaxseed is a rich source of lignans, which are dietary substances with many biologic functions, including cholesterol reduction. Additionally, flaxseed is one of the richest dietary sources of alpha-linolenic acid, which is also known to lower cholesterol. Scientists hypothesize that the reason whole or ground flaxseed is a better choice than flaxseed oil is the very high soluble-fiber content of both whole and ground flaxseed. The flaxseed shell is a rich source of soluble fiber, a substance known to favorably alter cholesterol levels.

The next logical question to ask is *how much* flaxseed you need to lower your cholesterol. Unfortunately, the answer is not crystal clear. Studies have used anywhere from 25 to 38 grams of whole or ground flaxseed. Just like plant stanol and sterol margarines, flaxseed provides both calories and fat. One level tablespoon of ground flaxseed (eight grams) provides 39 calories, 2.7 grams of fat, 2.2 grams of fiber, and 1.5 grams of protein. I generally encourage people to consume three to four tablespoons of flaxseed per day. This means up to 160 calories per day—just from flaxseed.

I usually suggest that a person try using between three and four tablespoons per day for a three-month period. At the end of that time period, I assess the effect it has had on the cholesterol. I ask how a person likes the taste, and how easy it has been to incorporate the flaxseed into his or her diet. If the response has been good, I always ask if it is something the person can imagine continuing for life. Just like any medication or supplement, flaxseed will only work if you continue to use it.

It is important to recognize that, although rare, flaxseed allergies can occur. Just as with peanut allergies, it is impossible to know who will develop an allergy and who will not. If you have never used flaxseed before, I recommend starting with a very small amount and making sure you are not alone when you use it for the first few times. This may sound overly cautious, but better safe than sorry. If you have multiple food allergies, it is probably best to discuss flaxseed with your allergist prior to using it.

Many large supermarkets sell flaxseed in bulk. It is also generally available at health-food stores. The whole seeds will keep well in your kitchen cabinet, stored in a glass jar or plastic container. However, ground flaxseed should be stored in the refrigerator, as it can become rancid. It should be used within one to two days of grinding. You can easily grind the seed in a small coffee grinder.

A study by Arjmandi and colleagues found that, in addition to its favorable impact on LDL cholesterol, whole or ground flaxseed can also lower another blood lipid called lipoprotein(a), also known as lp(a).

An elevated level of lipoprotein(a) is known to be a risk factor for the development of heart disease. A person can have an elevated LDL cholesterol level because of bad diet, bad genes, or some combination of the two; but an elevated lp(a) level is solely caused by bad genes. Lipoprotein(a) is an LDL-like particle with an attached protein called apoprotein(a). Just like LDL, lp(a) can clog up arteries. Lp(a) is actually worse than LDL because the apoprotein(a) confers an additional negative property — clotting. The apoprotein(a) looks very much like other clotting proteins, and it fools the body into thinking that it's one of our normal blood-clotting proteins.

People with high levels of lp(a) are at increased risk for developing heart disease because their lp(a) can clog up their arteries just like LDL. (In fact, lp(a) has been found in plaques within the heart arteries.) Having a high lp(a) level also increases the risk of clotting.

Most heart attacks are caused by the combination of a cholesterol deposit and a blood clot. When a cholesterol deposit within a heart artery cracks open, the inside of that deposit is exposed to blood flowing within the artery. The blood sees the inside of the deposit as "foreign," in other words, something that doesn't belong there. The natural response is to try to patch up the deposit with a blood clot (much like a scab on your knee). The problem with a blood clot on top of a cholesterol deposit is that it has the potential to completely block up a heart artery. If blood cannot flow freely through the heart artery, part of the heart muscle will be deprived of the nutrients and oxygen carried in the blood. That part of the heart muscle will die. This is called a heart attack. As you can see, an elevated lp(a) level can be quite deadly.

Fortunately, most people do not have levels of lp(a) high enough to get them into trouble. The average lp(a) level in the white population is between two and four mg/dl.

African-Americans tend to have somewhat higher levels (around 15 mg/dl). It is not until a person has a blood level of 20 to 30 mg/dl that cardiac risk accelerates.

Unfortunately, very few prescription medications lower lp(a). To date, niacin (which is a B vitamin), estrogen, and raloxifine (Evista) are the only commonly used drugs that positively impact lp(a). Until Arjmandi and colleagues found that 38 grams of whole or ground flaxseed (a little less than five tablespoons) could lower lp(a) by 7.4 percent, no other dietary measures had been shown to lower this lipoprotein. Theorists suggest that flaxseed contains some estrogenic compounds that lower lp(a).

As a rule, neither the medications just mentioned nor flaxseed are sufficient to fully normalize a person's lp(a) level. It is reassuring to note that data from the Familial Atherosclerosis Treatment Study (FATS) found that if LDL is dramatically lowered, lp(a) takes on less significance as a cardiac risk factor. In other words, in a person with very high lp(a) levels, the best bet is to dramatically lower the LDL. If LDL is lowered, lp(a) poses less of a cardiac risk.

26. Try Fish Oils

Fish oils are found in fish and other marine life, such as shrimp and lobster. Fish oils are a type of polyunsaturated fatty acids known as omega-3 or n-3 fatty acids. There are three different varieties of omega-3 fatty acids. Eicosapentenoic acid (EPA) and docosahexenoic acid (DHA) both exist in fish. The third variety of omega-3 fatty acid is alpha-linolenic acid (ALA), which is found not in fish but in soybeans, walnuts, and flaxseed.

In November of 2000, the American Heart Association published a revision of their dietary guidelines. The guidelines were revised because of (among other reasons) the growing body of information that suggests eating fish is good for a person's heart. The AHA now recommends that all Americans consume at least two three-ounce servings of fatty fish a week. Fatty fish, such as sardines, mackerel, herring, bluefish, salmon, and tuna, are preferred over leaner fish such as swordfish, red snapper, and sole because they contain much more of the omega-3 fatty acids that are believed to be the nutrients responsible for the cardiovascular benefits of fish.

One study to test the hypothesis that fish intake could alter cardiovascular outcome was the Diet and Reinfarction Trial (DART). DART was reported in 1989 in the *Lancet* (a prestigious British medical journal) and included 2,033 men who had recovered from a heart attack. After two years, the group of men who consumed fatty fish at least twice a week had 29 percent fewer deaths than the group of men who were not instructed to eat fish.

A second and much more recent study was published in 1999, also in the *Lancet.* This Italian study, called the GISSI-Prevenzione Study, included a total of 11,324 patients from 172 cardiac centers in Italy. At entry into the study, all participants had already suffered a heart attack. Patients were divided into four treatment groups. Group One received a single fish-oil capsule per day. Group Two received one vitamin E capsule per day. Group Three received both the fish-oil and vitamin E capsules. Group Four received neither the fish-oil nor the vitamin E capsules. At the end of three and a half years, persons treated with the fish-oil supplement had a dramatic reduction (between 15 and 20 percent) in death, heart attack, and stroke. Most striking was the 45 percent reduction in sudden cardiac death in those receiving fish oil. Vitamin E was not found in this study to provide any cardiovascular protection.

This information is enough to make anyone (except vegetarians) go out and eat fish or consider fish-oil supplements. The question is, *how* does fish oil protect against heart disease and stroke? The answer to this question is anything but simple. Fish oils appear to exert marked effects on our blood-clotting systems and a more modest impact on cholesterol; most striking is the ability of fish oils to lower triglyceride levels. Fish oils also appear to lower blood pressure slightly.

Although this book is about cholesterol, it is, in a larger sense, about maintaining a healthy heart. For this reason, I will digress a moment and address the impact of fish oils on clotting and how this might affect your heart. Although it is beyond the scope of this book to go into great scientific detail, it is important to point out that fish oils appear to influence our ability to form blood clots in many different ways. This includes affecting our platelets and clotting factors.

People such as Greenland Eskimos, who consume huge amounts of fatty fish, are known to have platelets that are less likely to clump together than the platelets of persons who consume a more typical American diet. Scientists speculate that this is one reason Eskimos have a low risk for developing cardiac disease. Remember that most heart attacks are caused by the combination of a cholesterol deposit and a blood clot. Platelets are the blood-clotting cells, so making them less sticky (less likely to clump together) is likely to reduce the risk of a heart attack.

Fish oils have also been shown to increase the blood level of tissue plasminogen activator (TPA). This is the same substance we give to patients in the emergency room when they come in having a heart attack. It is also known as a "clot buster." TPA is a natural clot-dissolving substance. We all have some TPA in our bloodstream; however, it appears that people who eat lots of fish have greater amounts of TPA than people who don't.

Still other studies have shown that people who eat fish regularly have lower blood levels of fibrinogen and Factor VIII (two substances which promote blood clots).

What about cholesterol? Although fish oils appear to have a modest impact on total cholesterol, and possibly can raise HDL cholesterol (the good cholesterol) slightly, in my practice the major role of fish oils is as a triglyceride-lowering agent.

Although it is possible to estimate the impact of a given amount of fish oil on triglyceride levels for an entire population, in any individual the impact of a given dose of fish oil cannot be predicted. In a study that included 50 participants, all of whom had high cholesterol, Adler and Holub reported that 3.6 grams of omega-3 fatty acids resulted in a 37.3 percent reduction in triglycerides. The participants in this study were also found to experience a 9 percent increase in HDL cholesterol and an 8.5 percent increase in LDL cholesterol. This LDL-cholesterol–raising effect has been seen in some, but not all, studies.

One of the difficulties in interpreting fish-oil studies is that in studies where fish oils are used to replace saturated fats in the diet, LDL cholesterol seems to fall. When the fish oil is added to the diet and the amount of saturated fat remains the same, LDL cholesterol level either remains the same or increases slightly.

Overall, it appears that fish-oil capsules can be useful in lowering triglycerides. They are particularly useful in individuals with markedly elevated triglycerides (over 500 mg/dl). It should be pointed out that not all fish-oil capsules are created equal. A 1,000-mg capsule can contain anywhere from 300 to 500 mg of omega-3 fatty acids. There are some 2,000-mg capsules that contain almost 900 mg of omega-3 fatty acids. It is also important to recognize that fish oil contains calories. If you decide to give fish oils a try, you should see a change in your triglycerides within four weeks.

In our clinic, we ask people to gradually increase their intake of fish-oil capsules to a maximum of between five and ten capsules per day. We specifically ask people to gradually increase their intake so as to minimize the most troublesome side effect (burping and fishy breath). I have found that taking fish-oil capsules with dinner (or a person's largest meal) also minimizes this side effect. In general, we ask people to use the schedule in Table 8:

TABLE 8 Recommended Dosage of Fish-Oil Capsules

Week	Dose
One	One capsule
Two	Two capsules
Three	Three capsules
Four	Four capsules
Five	Five capsules

We have our patients remain at the five-capsule dose for four to six weeks and then we recheck their lipid profile. The dose of fish oil is adjusted based on the triglyceride response or on side effects.

Rose is a woman who was referred to us because she had side effects with every cholesterol medication her doctor had tried her on. She had an astronomical triglyceride level. When we met, her lipids looked like this:

Rose's Level	Desirable Level
Total cholesterol 264 mg/dl	< 200 mg/dl
Triglycerides 501 mg/dl	< 150 mg/dl
LDL cholesterol [could not calculate]	< 130 mg/dl
HDL cholesterol 48 mg/dl	> 45 mg/dl

Rose is a nurse, and she was doing all the right things: no alcohol, very little sugar, no fruit juice or soda. She was walking two and a half miles a day. Although this had served to lower her triglycerides from a high of 950 mg/dl, she clearly needed to lower them further. We decided to try fish-oil capsules. She gradually worked up to seven capsules with the following result:

Rose's Level	Desirable Level
Total cholesterol 230 mg/dl	< 200 mg/dl
Triglycerides 205 mg/dl	< 150 mg/dl
LDL cholesterol 143 mg/dl	< 130 mg/dl
HDL cholesterol 46 mg/dl	> 45 mg/dl

At this point, we were thrilled (but not totally satisfied). When I first met Rose, I could not measure her LDL cholesterol—if triglycerides are over 400 mg/dl, LDL is difficult to determine. Now that we could measure her LDL, we could see it needed a little work. I recommended adding two tablespoons of Benecol Light (previously mentioned). Hesitantly, I also asked if she could bump her fish-oil intake to nine capsules. She agreed to both. Rose explained that although she didn't like the number of fish-oil capsules she was taking, she was glad to have finally found something she could take without side effects.

Her lipid profile eight weeks later looked like this:

Rose's Level	Desirable Level
Total cholesterol 192 mg/dl	< 200 mg/dl
Triglycerides 175 mg/dl	< 150 mg/dl
LDL cholesterol 106 mg/dl	< 130 mg/dl
HDL cholesterol 51 mg/dl	> 45 mg/dl

We decided we were satisfied. Over the last year, Rose has remained on this same program. Her triglycerides have ranged from a low of 145 mg/dl to a high of 200 mg/dl. The 200 mg/dl reading occurred in December; I'll let you guess the cause. One final note on Rose: when we first met, her blood pressure was 144/92 mmHg. On the fish-oil capsules (which are known to have a slight impact on blood pressure) her blood pressure now is routinely 132/80 mmHg.

If you decide to try fish-oil capsules, it is crucial for you to discuss your plan with your doctor. As I pointed out earlier, one of the ways fish oils work is by preventing blood clots. While this can be beneficial in some circumstances, it can also cause a person to bruise more easily and possibly develop nosebleeds, or even more serious bleeding complications. Fish-oil supplementation is not recommended for pregnant women. I do not suggest fish-oil supplements for children.

27. Talk to Your Doctor About Guggulipid

Guggulipid is the resin or sap from *Commiphora mukul* (the mukul myrrh tree). The mukul myrrh tree, which grows in

India, is really more of a shrub. As early as 1971, the positive effects of guggulipid (also known as gugulipid, guggul and guggulu) on cholesterol were reported by Kapoor and colleagues in the proceedings of the Seminar on Disorders of Lipid Metabolism, held in New Delhi, India.

The active ingredients in guggulipid appear to be two plant steroids called Z-guggulsterone and E-guggulsterone. In an elegant study by Singh and colleagues, these two steroids were shown to increase the uptake of LDL cholesterol by the liver. This, in turn, significantly lowers the LDL cholesterol level in the bloodstream. Guggulipid has been shown to lower both LDL cholesterol (by about 12 percent) and triglycerides (by about 15 percent). Some studies have even shown some HDL improvement with guggulipid.

Guggulipid is used extensively in Ayurvedic medicine. Ayurvedic medicine uses drugs extracted from herbs, as well as diet, massage, meditation, and exercise, to treat disease. In India, guggulipid is sold as a drug, whereas in the United States it is available in health-food stores. The typical dose of guggulipid is 25 mg three times a day with meals.

Most people have no side effects with guggulipid. Some people, however, have reported mild nausea, diarrhea, and headaches. Generally, these mild side effects resolve with continued use. If you choose to use guggulipid, I think it is essential for you to let your doctor know. While it appears that the literature on guggulipid is solid science, the studies have typically been small. It is possible that guggulipid has side effects that have not yet been determined.

This being said, I must tell you that I do have a number of patients who have used guggulipid with excellent success. In fact, one of my patients, Dr. Edna Katz (a psychotherapist), introduced me to guggulipid. She has been on it for almost a decade without adverse side effects.

Suzanne, a patient who sees my partner, did a guggulipid experiment: we measured her cholesterol profile on and off guggulipid, for a total of four times. We first measured her baseline cholesterol levels; she then took guggulipid for three months and we rechecked her cholesterol profile. She came off the guggulipid for three months, we rechecked her lipid profile, and she then went back on the guggulipid and we checked her values once again. Here are her levels:

No Guggulipid

Suzanne's Level	*Desirable Level*
Total cholesterol 280 mg/dl	< 200 mg/dl
Triglycerides 78 mg/dl	< 150 mg/dl
LDL cholesterol 182 mg/dl	< 130 mg/dl
HDL cholesterol 83 mg/dl	> 45 mg/dl

Guggulipid (25 mg three times a day)

Suzanne's Level	*Desirable Level*
Total cholesterol 244 mg/dl	< 200 mg/dl
Triglycerides 65 mg/dl	< 150 mg/dl
LDL cholesterol 137 mg/dl	< 130 mg/dl
HDL cholesterol 94 mg/dl	> 45 mg/dl

Back Off Guggulipid

Suzanne's Level	*Desirable Level*
Total cholesterol 275 mg/dl	< 200 mg/dl
Triglycerides 70 mg/dl	< 150 mg/dl
LDL cholesterol 181 mg/dl	< 130 mg/dl
HDL cholesterol 80 mg/dl	> 45 mg/dl

Guggulipid (25 mg three times a day) and Ground Flaxseed (2 tablespoons per day)

Suzanne's Level	Desirable Level
Total cholesterol 208 mg/dl	< 200 mg/dl
Triglycerides 54 mg/dl	< 150 mg/dl
LDL cholesterol 117 mg/dl	< 130 mg/dl
HDL cholesterol 80 mg/dl	> 45 mg/dl

While the addition of flaxseed during the last cycle makes it a little difficult to determine the exact impact of the guggulipid, the impact appears substantial nonetheless. Her liver functions remained stable throughout the course of the experiment.

All told, we probably have 12 patients in our practice on guggulipid. A number of the 12 are taking many other "nutraceuticals," so the impact of guggulipid is difficult to gauge. If you decide to use guggulipid, you can probably expect at least a 10 to 15 percent reduction in LDL cholesterol and perhaps a reduction in triglycerides as well. Remember to consult your doctor before beginning any herbal medicines.

28. Rethink Garlic and Lecithin

Reports in the medical literature over the past 25 years have suggested that oral garlic supplements might be effective in reducing cholesterol. These studies often found as much as a 15 percent reduction in cholesterol with various preparations and doses of garlic. Based on these studies (which I must say were often small and poorly designed), I used to recommend garlic to my patients. My feeling was that garlic might help and certainly has no side effects (with the exception of the bad-breath issue).

In 1998, two studies published within a week of each other changed my practice. Dr. Jonathan Isaacsohn, Dr. Marvin Moser and Dr. Evan Stein reported the first trial in the *Archives of Internal Medicine*. This study was very well-designed. The 50 participants all had elevated cholesterol levels. Twenty-eight people received the garlic preparation called Kwai (300 mg three times a day). The remaining 22 participants received an identical placebo. Cholesterol values were drawn at baseline and after 12 weeks of therapy. Neither group experienced any change in cholesterol values.

One week later, Berthold and colleagues published similar findings in the *Journal of the American Medical Association* (*JAMA*). This trial was a bit smaller (25 participants) and used a different garlic preparation, garlic oil (5 mg twice a day for 12 weeks). Again, all subjects had high cholesterol levels. Half the participants received the garlic preparation, and half received a matching placebo for 12 weeks. Study subjects subsequently took nothing for four weeks (a washout period) and then switched (for 12 weeks) to whichever therapy they did not have during the first 12 weeks. Participants' cholesterol levels were not altered by the garlic.

These well-designed studies certainly cast some doubt on the garlic-cholesterol hypothesis. Some people have criticized these studies, saying that only *fresh* garlic will work to lower cholesterol.

Very recently (September 2000), Clare Stevinson published a meta-analysis of all garlic trials in the *Annals of Internal Medicine*. This analysis concluded that garlic *might* be superior to placebo in reducing cholesterol levels, but that the size of the effect is quite small.

It is certainly possible that garlic may have other health benefits, but in my opinion garlic should be eaten because you like the taste — not as a cholesterol-lowering therapy.

When patients come in for their first visit to my office, frequently they are already taking lots of different dietary supplements. Lecithin is one very common supplement. Most patients I see are taking it because they have heard it is a "fat emulsifier" and will therefore lower their cholesterol. They go on to explain that they believe lecithin will dissolve the fat and cholesterol in their blood and render it harmless. Perhaps if lecithin made it into the bloodstream, this would be possible. In fact, the lecithin a person takes as an oral supplement is destroyed in the stomach and never makes it into the blood. Although lecithin is not particularly expensive, it is not a worthwhile way to spend your money. I certainly do not recommend it as a cholesterol-lowering agent.

PART FOUR

Exercise

29. Develop an Exercise Program

At the Cholesterol Management Center, we view exercise as essential. Most people who come to work with us not only need to lower their cholesterol, they need to lose weight as well. It has been my experience that anyone can lose weight and lower his or her cholesterol with a diet. However, if one wants to *maintain* that weight loss and cholesterol reduction, exercise is essential.

You may be asking yourself, "How much exercise is enough?" If your goal is cholesterol reduction and weight loss, you should really plan for daily exercise. The American Heart Association recommends that all Americans burn 2,000 calories a week exercising. This translates into walking three miles a day. But while this should be your goal, any exercise is better than no exercise. It is also important to remember that Rome wasn't built in a day. Don't expect to go from being a couch potato to walking three miles a day. The program outlined a bit later in this chapter will help you work up to walking three miles a day.

Say you are lean, with no need to lose weight, but you have a high cholesterol count nonetheless. You want to know what the least amount of time is that you can exercise and still get cardiovascular benefit and cholesterol reduction. The short answer is three days a week, 30 minutes per session (more in a moment regarding intensity). However, even if you don't need to lose weight, you are likely to get a greater cholesterol benefit if you exercise on a daily basis.

Before you begin any exercise routine, I urge you to consult your physician. He or she knows your case best. Your doctor may recommend that you undergo a stress test prior to beginning a program. Not only does a stress test help your physician determine if exercise will be safe for you, it also allows him or her to give you a prescription for exercise.

Intuitively, we all know that exercise is an important part of a healthy lifestyle. Most people remember a time in their life when exercise wasn't a chore but a delight. It is hard to know what happened to the person who loved running around the school yard playing tag or was happy to play basketball for hours on end. For most people, the transformation is insidious; it begins in high school. If a boy or girl doesn't play on an organized school or town team, daily structured activity generally goes by the wayside. People who participate in high-school athletics typically hang it up at graduation. The fact that the average American gains about a pound a year after completing his or her formal education is directly related to the development of a sedentary lifestyle. The reduction in energy expenditure and the weight gain each contribute independently to the age-related rise in cholesterol that is typically seen in industrialized societies.

Countries in which life demands a significant amount of daily physical activity do not experience the marked increase in cholesterol noted in the United States. It is therefore only logical to speculate that an increase in physical activity might lower cholesterol.

You are probably also wondering how much improvement you are likely to see in your cholesterol profile as a result of your new exercise program. Exercise impacts HDL cholesterol and triglyceride levels most dramatically. While LDL cholesterol can improve with vigorous physical activity, the impact is generally not dramatic.

As you might guess, a person's baseline cholesterol profile also influences the magnitude of change that can be expected. What do I mean by this? Let's examine some data collected at the Ochsner Heart and Vascular Institute in New Orleans and the Massachusetts General Hospital in Boston. Drs. Carl Lavie and Richard Milani examined the impact of a 12-week exercise program on 591 cardiac patients. Patients exercised for one hour (10-minute warm-up, 40-minute exercise program, followed by a 10-minute cooldown) three times a week in a supervised setting. Exercise intensity was individually designed for each patient so that the patient's heart rate was between 75 and 85 percent of his or her maximum heart rate. (MHR will be explained in a moment.) Participants were also encouraged to exercise on their own at least once, but preferably three times, per week. Cholesterol levels were measured at baseline and at the completion of the 12-week program.

Changes in cholesterol profiles were strongly dependent on baseline cholesterol levels. This study reported specifically on the 243 out of 591 participants who had low baseline HDL cholesterol levels (defined in this study as less than or equal to 35 mg/dl). Overall exercise in this group resulted in a 12 percent increase in HDL cholesterol and a 14 percent drop in triglycerides, but only a 1 percent drop in LDL cholesterol.

To sort this out further, the authors decided to look at the lipid changes in participants with low HDL cholesterol (again defined as a level below 35 mg/dl) and normal triglycerides (defined as below 150 mg/dl). In this population, HDL cholesterol rose by 9 percent, triglycerides rose by 4 percent, and LDL cholesterol fell by 3 percent.

On the other hand, participants with low HDL cholesterol (below 35 mg/dl) who had elevated triglycerides (above 250 mg/dl) could expect an 11 percent increase in HDL cholesterol, a 22 percent fall in triglycerides, and a 9 percent rise in LDL.

In summary, in people with low HDL cholesterol, exercise can be expected to increase this lipid by about 10 percent. Similar increases have been noted in people with normal baseline HDL levels (i.e. above 45 mg/dl). With regard to triglycerides, the data is very clear: people with high triglycerides may experience significant improvement (between a 20 and 25 percent fall) with vigorous activity. The LDL-cholesterol–lowering impact of exercise is limited (about 2 to 3 percent). However, if exercise results in weight loss, we can often see a much more dramatic fall in LDL cholesterol levels (10 to 15 percent). In this situation, it is really the weight loss and not the exercise that causes the improvement in LDL cholesterol. But from a practical point of view, this doesn't really matter. The important thing is that the cholesterol improves.

As you plan out your exercise program, keep three things in mind: frequency, intensity, and time. This is also known as the F.I.T. principle.

Frequency

In the previous paragraphs, we explored the issue of how frequently a person needs to exercise. Ultimately, how frequently you exercise will depend on your fitness goals. If you have never exercised before, it is important to start off slowly. Even if your goal is weight loss, starting out with only three exercise sessions a week gets you started and achieves a conditioning effect, but prevents burnout. If weight loss is your goal, you will ultimately need to double the frequency to a minimum of six (and better yet, seven) times a week.

Intensity

To make the most of your exercise program, it is important to work at the proper intensity. Intensity is really how hard you are pushing yourself. You want to be working hard enough to achieve a training effect, to turn fat into muscle, but not so hard that you kick your body into anaerobic metabolism.

How can you tell if you are exercising at the proper intensity? One way is by checking your pulse and determining your target heart rate. You can check your pulse in any number of locations (your neck, wrist, behind your knee, on your foot). Your pulse is simply your heart rate. Each beat of your heart creates a pulse that you can feel and count. One of the easiest places to check your pulse is at your wrist. Place your index and middle fingers on the thumb side of your wrist. Here you will feel your radial pulse. Count the number of pulses over a ten-second period and multiply this number by six to get your pulse-per-minute rate. Your heart rate (the number of times your heart beats per minute) is an indirect measurement of how hard you are exercising. The target heart rate (THR) range is a common method of measuring exercise intensity.

First, figure your maximum heart rate using the following formula:

220 − your age = maximum heart rate (MHR)

Example: a 50-year-old male or female:
220 − 50 = 170 beats per minute

In order to lower your cholesterol and achieve physical fitness, it is not necessary to work out at your maximum heart rate. In fact, this would be undesirable, especially as you begin a regular exercise program. Studies have determined that exercising at a heart rate of between 50 and 85 percent of your maximum heart rate is sufficient to produce excellent results and a training effect. Here is an example of the equations to use to determine the THR, with the same 50-year-old man or woman:

170 × 0.50 = 85 beats per minute
170 × 0.85 = 145 beats per minute

The THR range is therefore 85 to 145 beats per minute.

Table 9 will help you determine your own target heart rate and 10-second pulse rate:

TABLE 9 Target Heart Rates

Age	Maximum HR	Target HR	10-Second Pulse
20	200	100–170	17–28
25	195	98–166	17–28
30	190	95–162	16–27

Age	Maximum HR	Target HR	10-Second Pulse
35	185	92–157	16–27
40	180	90–153	15–26
45	175	88–149	15–26
50	170	85–145	14–25
55	165	82–140	14–25
60	160	80–136	13–24
65	155	78–131	13–24
70	150	75–128	12–23
75	145	72–123	12–23
80	140	70–119	11–22

Some people have a great deal of difficulty measuring their pulse. This does not mean that these people should not exercise — or if they do, that they will not be able to accurately assess the intensity of their program. The "talk test" is by far the easiest (and a fairly accurate) method of determining whether a person is exercising at the appropriate intensity to achieve aerobic fitness. As the name "talk test" implies, you should be able to talk as you are exercising without huffing and puffing excessively. On the other hand, you should be winded enough that you shouldn't be able to deliver the Gettysburg Address. If you can, you need to push a little harder.

Time

The issue of time has already been partially addressed. Clearly, you want to spend enough time on your exercise program to achieve cardiovascular fitness and improve your cholesterol level. The bare minimum is 30 minutes three times a week (this does not include warm-up and cooldown times). But for most of my patients who are hoping for weight loss, three times a week is not enough. If you want to lose weight, you must generally exercise for 45 to 60 minutes per day if you choose an exercise like walking and about 30 minutes per day if you choose a higher-intensity exercise like a stair stepper, jogging/running, Nordic track, kick-boxing, or a spin class.

Some people who are either short on time or have difficulty exercising for a full 45 to 60 minutes ask me if it is possible to do several shorter sessions over the course of the day. There is mounting evidence that a few short exercise sessions during a day provide a person with the same cholesterol and weight-loss benefits as one long session. This knowledge allows a person to begin an exercise program of short sessions and progress just as quickly as someone who is doing long sessions less frequently.

Now that you are ready to begin an exercise program, it's important to plan it out. But remember nothing needs to be set in stone. The American College of Sports Medicine (ACSM) defines three stages for an aerobic exercise program. The stages are an initial conditioning stage, an improvement stage, and a final, or maintenance, stage, which is meant to last a lifetime.

The ACSM also provides guidelines regarding the expected rate of progress. Remember, these are only guidelines. It is generally recommended that the initial conditioning stage last four to six weeks. The improvement stage lasts anywhere between 12 and 24 weeks, and the maintenance stage lasts a lifetime. Many people continue to become more fit even during the maintenance stage, and it is during this stage that they may attempt new types of exercises. People who enjoy a challenge may consider training for a road race or bike race.

As you progress through the stages, remember that the recommended rate of progress varies from individual to individual. Some people will get bored with the initial conditioning stage and will want to move on to the improvement stage within two weeks, whereas others might spend 12 to 16 weeks working on the initial conditioning stage. Neither approach is wrong. Ultimately, you know your body best. I remind you that it is important to discuss any new exercise program and your plans for progress with your physician.

30. Condition Your Body

During the initial conditioning stage of your exercise program, two things are crucial: consistency and patience. You will not improve if you only exercise once a week. Conversely, if you jump into an exercise program and try to work out seven days a week for 60 minutes per session, you may well experience an overuse injury. I suggest the program in Table 10:

TABLE 10
Suggested Exercise Program—Conditioning Stage

Weeks	Frequency	Intensity	Time
1–2	3–5 times a week	50–60 percent MHR	15 minutes
3–4	3–5 times a week	50–60 percent MHR	15–18 minutes
5–6	3–5 times a week	50–60 percent MHR	18–20 minutes

MHR = Maximum Heart Rate.
Your target heart rate is 50 to 60 percent of the MHR.

I suggest trying to push for five times a week if you know your goal is weight loss. If your only goal is cholesterol reduction, then three times a week for up to 20 minutes per session is sufficient at this stage. Table 11 gives you your target heart-rate range for the initial conditioning stage:

TABLE 11 Target Heart Rates—Conditioning Stage

Age	50–60 Percent MHR	10-Second Pulse
20	100–120	17–20
25	98–117	17–20
30	95–114	16–19
35	92–111	16–19
40	90–108	15–18
45	88–105	15–18
50	85–102	14–17
55	82–99	14–17
60	80–96	13–16
65	78–93	13–16
70	75–90	12–15
75	72–87	12–15
80	70–84	11–14
85	68–81	11–14

31. Improve Your Fitness Level

You are now ready to move to the improvement stage. On average, this stage will last between 12 and 24 weeks. Again, you decide how quickly to progress. Table 12 gives my recommendations:

TABLE 12
Suggested Exercise Program—Improvement Stage

Weeks	Frequency	Intensity	Time
7–10	4–5 times a week	60–70 percent MHR	20 minutes
11–14	4–5 times a week	70–80 percent MHR	25 minutes
15–20	5–6 times a week	70–85 percent MHR	30 minutes
21–25	6–7 times a week	70–85 percent MHR	45–60 minutes

During the improvement stage, it is up to you to determine your goals. If weight loss is important to you, I suggest gradually working up to a frequency of six to seven sessions per week. If cholesterol improvement is your only concern, you may continue to exercise only three times a week during this stage. However, it is likely you will get a greater cholesterol benefit if you push yourself to do six or seven sessions per week. Likewise, let your body guide you regarding intensity. It is perfectly acceptable to continue at 50 to 60 percent of the MHR during the improvement stage. Finally, almost everyone should aim to accumulate 30 minutes of exercise each day they exercise. This does not have to occur all at once—it might be accomplished as two 15-minute sessions or three 10-minute sessions. Again, if weight loss is an objective, the goal should be to accumulate between 45 and 60 minutes nearly every day. Here are the target heart rates for the improvement stage:

TABLE 13 Target Heart Rates—Improvement Stage

Age	60–85 Percent MHR	10-Second Pulse
20	120–170	20–28
25	117–166	20–28
30	114–162	19–27
35	111–157	19–27
40	108–153	18–26
45	105–149	18–26
50	102–145	17–25
55	99–140	17–25
60	96–136	16–24
65	93–131	16–24
70	90–128	15–23
75	87–123	15–23
80	84–119	14–22
85	81–115	14–22

32. Maintain Your Fitness Level

The maintenance stage requires persistence and commitment. You have acquired the skills necessary to maintain an exercise program for life. Staying committed is now the challenge.

Some people find that working with a partner sustains enthusiasm. Other people reward themselves with a prize if they accumulate a certain number of miles per month. Charting mileage is fun. One of my patients set a year-long goal to walk 1,000 miles. She figured out where she would end up if she traveled 1,000 miles south from her home and pretended to be walking there; she plotted her weekly progress on a AAA map. At the end of the year, she and her husband flew there for a vacation. They had a great time telling their story to people in St. Augustine, Florida. Another way to stay excited about exercise is to train for a worthy cause. You can participate in the American Heart Association Walk or some other charitable event.

Finally, depending upon where you live in this country, you must plan how you will continue to maintain your exercise program during the winter months. Many people invest in a treadmill. This is an excellent idea, but always purchase an electric treadmill. Self-propelled treadmills are very difficult to work with and, as a result, people give up.

Why a treadmill? Zeni and colleagues evaluated four different indoor exercise machines (treadmill, cross-country skiing simulator, rowing machine, and stair stepper) and found that the treadmill resulted in the greatest energy expenditure. If the treadmill doesn't excite you, consider joining a gym in the winter. Still others walk at a local mall or high school. Many malls or high schools open early to accommodate walkers.

In general, during the maintenance stage you should plan on walking six or seven times a week at 70 to 85 percent of your MHR. Each session should last about 60 minutes. Again, you can customize this according to your fitness goals.

33. Be Sure to Warm Up and Cool Down

Because you will want to continue your exercise program for the rest of your life, it is crucial to take steps to avoid injury. Performing a warm-up and cooldown are two very important components of your exercise program. For many people who want to jump right into their exercise routine, this can seem tedious. I assure you, they are essential.

The warm-up consists of a five-to-ten minute period of either stretching or a less intense version of whatever your chosen exercise is. I generally recommend a slow walk. This slow walk allows your body to reach your target heart rate (whatever it may be) safely and comfortably.

The cooldown helps slow your heart down gradually. Over the course of a five-to-ten-minute slow walk, you should be able to bring your heart rate fairly close to your pre-exercise heart rate. Slowing your heart rate gradually helps prevent blood from pooling in your legs, greatly reducing the risk of fainting and lightheadedness. Stretching is also a good idea during the cooldown phase of your program.

Remember, the warm-up and cooldown phases of your exercise session do not count toward total time exercised. If you are aiming for a 60-minute program, the warm-up and cooldown can add between 10 and 20 minutes.

34. Be Patient with Yourself!

As you embark on an exercise program, it is important to be patient with yourself. You may not have enjoyed exercise in the past, but if you give yourself eight weeks to get into the improvement stage, you will find that your body can do more than you ever thought it could. You will become proud of what you have accomplished. You will hate to admit it, but you will begin to enjoy walking (or biking or swimming—whatever exercise you have chosen).

Even if you don't quite get to the point of liking exercise, consider this: One of my patients told me, "There is nothing like having exercised." After a year of regular exercise, he still didn't enjoy the program, but he knew he needed to exercise and was committed to doing so. He told me he routinely exercised first thing in the morning so that he could get it over with and could start his day with the good and satisfying feeling of "having already exercised."

I hope exercise will be more enjoyable to you than it is for my patient, but no matter how you accomplish it, exercise is crucial to cardiovascular fitness. It certainly has a positive impact on cholesterol levels (especially HDL cholesterol and triglycerides). The degree to which LDL cholesterol improves with exercise is largely dependent on the amount of weight lost as a result of exercise. Why not head out today to buy a good pair of walking shoes? That's all you need to get started on the trip toward better health.

PART FIVE

Quit Smoking

35. Understand the Effects of Smoking on Cholesterol

Cigarette smoking has an adverse impact on a person's cholesterol profile; it dramatically lowers a person's HDL cholesterol. In the Framingham Offspring Study, Garrison and colleagues found that in women, smoking lowers the protective (HDL) cholesterol by about 6 mg/dl. In men, smokers have an HDL cholesterol level that is 4 mg/dl lower than their nonsmoking peers.

If a drop in HDL cholesterol of this magnitude doesn't impress you, consider this: For every 1 mg/dl increase in HDL, there is a corresponding 2 percent decrease in cardiac risk in men and a 3 percent decrease in women. If the average woman increases her HDL cholesterol by 6 mg/dl when she quits smoking, she can expect an 18 percent reduction in cardiac risk. And because the average man will increase his HDL cholesterol by 4 mg/dl when he quits smoking, he can expect an 8 percent reduction in cardiac risk. But because quitting cigarette smoking has so many other positive effects (read on), the cardiac risk reduction is actually much greater than 8 or 18 percent. By cardiac risk I mean risk of a heart event (heart attack, bypass surgery, angioplasty).

Compared to nonsmokers, smokers have highly oxidized LDL cholesterol particles. What is oxidation, and how does it impact the LDL cholesterol? When an LDL cholesterol particle undergoes the process of oxidation, it becomes chemically modified. Once oxidized, LDL cholesterol particles become smaller, which one would normally think is a good thing. However, small LDL cholesterol particles have a very easy time getting into the artery wall and setting up shop. Oxidized LDL cholesterol particles are the main component of a cholesterol plaque, which can block the heart arteries and predispose a person to a heart attack.

Within two weeks of quitting smoking, a person may experience an improvement in HDL cholesterol. His or her LDL cholesterol is less likely to be oxidized. By six months, the HDL cholesterol is back to baseline (pre-smoking level), and the LDL cholesterol is no longer oxidized.

Cholesterol isn't the only thing adversely impacted by smoking. Each time you light up, you increase your heart rate, decrease your heart's ability to carry and deliver oxygen, and activate your platelets (the blood-clotting cells). As we discussed earlier in this book, heart attacks generally occur when a cholesterol deposit in a heart artery cracks open and is topped with a blood clot. The combination of a cholesterol deposit and blood clot leads to the complete blockage of a heart artery. Because smoking cigarettes adversely impacts both sides of the equation, quitting is one of the most important things you will ever do!

36. Quit Smoking

So how do you go about quitting? Let me say from the outset, quitting smoking is one of the hardest things you will ever do, but it will also be one of the most rewarding. Without even meeting you, I can say you are probably fed up with the habit yourself. The fact is, at least 80 percent of adult smokers desperately want to quit. Some people are able to quit when faced with the health consequences of their habit, but for most people the information just makes them feel worse — not more resolved.

You *can* become a nonsmoker. It won't be easy, but there are things you can do to make the road a little smoother. An important first step is to find out just how addicted you are. To determine this, answer these questions: Do you smoke within half an hour of waking up in the morning? Do you smoke more than a pack of cigarettes a day?

Studies have shown that smokers who need that first morning cigarette are the most highly addicted. Because the level of nicotine in your bloodstream declines dramatically as you sleep, highly addicted people "need" a cigarette the minute they wake in the morning. This sends the level of nicotine in the bloodstream up and allows the smoker to start his or her day. If this is your situation, you can still become a nonsmoker, but it will be more difficult for you than it will be for a person who can wait until noon before having a cigarette. (It's important to know this so you can avoid comparing yourself with a friend who quit with no difficulty.)

The second question is fairly straightforward. People who smoke more than a pack a day tend to be more highly addicted than those who smoke only a few cigarettes a day.

In general, I suggest that people who need to smoke first thing in the morning and people who smoke more than a pack a day strongly consider using a smoking cessation aid. This may be the oral medication bupropion (also known as Zyban or Wellbutrin), or a nicotine gum, patch, nasal spray, or inhaler. A smoking-cessation support group or structured class can also be very helpful.

Now that you have assessed your level of addiction, it is also important to assess your motivation to quit. You can probably list a host of reasons for quitting. Your blood pressure will go down. Your protective cholesterol (the HDL or high-density lipoprotein cholesterol) will go up. You will decrease your risk of heart disease, stroke, bladder cancer, and lung cancer. You are much less likely to develop chronic lung disease. You will improve your ability to exercise. Your self-esteem will rise. Your children, spouse, or significant other will be proud of you. You won't have to spend another winter standing outside your office building with all the other banished smokers. You will get a break on life insurance. You will smell better. Food will taste better. Your ceilings will not need to be painted as frequently.

Whatever your motivating force, it is important that you are very committed because there will be lots of tough moments, especially in the first month. This is the most difficult time because you have not only the physical symptoms of withdrawal to contend with, but the psychological as well. After a month, all the unpleasant withdrawal symptoms (irritability, trouble sleeping, difficulty concentrating, cough, constipation, chest pain, and shakiness) are gone. "Only" the psychological addiction remains. This is why some smokers report still wanting a cigarette years after quitting.

One of my patients tried at least a dozen times to quit smoking and has now been off cigarettes for four years. He told me that every time he gets the urge for a cigarette (for him it is always at a restaurant after a very satisfying meal), he tries to remember how tough that first month off cigarettes was for him and his family. Not wanting to relive that month is his motivation. I think he is only half-joking when he says his wife would divorce him if she had to go through another month like that.

Once you are highly motivated, you are ready for the next step — setting a quit date. Ideally you should give yourself two weeks to prepare. You will spend the first week looking at your current smoking habits. Although you might want to cut back during this week, I generally advise people to simply record every cigarette they smoke. Attach an index card to your package of cigarettes. Each time you smoke a cigarette, write down the time of day and what you were doing. It is also helpful to note how badly you wanted the cigarette. At the end of seven days, look at your seven index cards. Do any patterns emerge? Do you smoke more when you are stressed? Bored? Tired? Hungry? After meals? With alcohol? With coffee or tea? What cigarettes do you want the most, and what cigarettes are purely out of habit? Pick out the five cigarettes you want most per day.

For the next week, smoke only those five. You should also spend this week getting ready for the new you:

- Tell your friends and family when you will become a nonsmoker.
- Practice sitting in the nonsmoking section of a restaurant.
- Stock up on sugar-free hard candies and sugar-free freeze pops.
- Pick up a few jigsaw puzzles.
- Buy yourself a new low-stress computer game.
- Enroll in a night course requiring you to use your hands (woodworking, painting, quilting).
- Get out your old board games and find a nonsmoking partner.
- Stock up on herbal teas and bubble bath.
- Buy a few new relaxing CDs.
- Declare your home a smoke-free zone as of your quit date.
- Toss out your ashtrays.
- Clean out all the ashtrays in your car. Fill them up with cinnamon-flavored toothpicks.
- Have your car detailed so that it smells clean and fresh.
- Have your drapes and carpets cleaned.

Now you are ready! I recommend that you quit smoking on a Saturday or a day off. Try to plan a very relaxed day for your first day as a nonsmoker. It will be helpful for you to plan a day of smoke-free activities: go to a movie, go to the library, go for a long walk. Tell your friends and family that you are quitting cigarettes and ask for their help and encouragement.

The first four weeks off cigarettes are the hardest. You are likely to be irritable and anxious, especially when you get the urge to smoke. Those first few weeks you will no doubt spend a great deal of time thinking about cigarettes; many people even dream about them. An intense craving for a cigarette is a signal to hold on tight and recognize what is happening; intense cravings only last a couple of minutes.

During that time try:

- Going for a walk or a bike ride
- Brushing your teeth
- Taking ten deep breaths in through your nose and letting them out slowly through your mouth
- Sucking on sugar-free hard candy
- Drinking a glass of water
- Calling a friend

Just a few more words on how you might feel during your first few weeks as a nonsmoker. Aside from feeling irritable, many of my patients complain that they feel washed out and extremely tired, but unable to sleep well. Many also mention that instead of getting rid of their smoker's cough, it has actually gotten worse. All of these are common and will get better.

Nicotine is a stimulant, so it makes sense that when your body is abruptly cut off you might feel very tired. But why should you have trouble sleeping? The answer to this is less clear, but it appears that nicotine has a strong influence over sleep patterns and that abrupt withdrawal can cause marked insomnia—even in people who feel very tired and want to sleep. The insomnia tends to be short-lived, generally no longer than a week or so.

The reason the smoker's cough increases is that the cilia (small filamentous tubules that line healthy lung passages), which have been destroyed by years of smoking, quickly begin to grow back (more hopeful evidence of the body's ability to heal itself!). As they do, a cough can develop. In fact, this itself can help get rid of some of the residual debris that has built up in the lungs over years of smoking. The cough is typically very short-lived.

Many people also tell me that when they quit smoking they suddenly developed constipation. At first I didn't really pay much attention to this complaint, but after hearing it a few times I went to the medical literature and found that it is true. This is the last thing you need to add to your list of problems as you quit smoking, so be proactive. Increase exercise as you quit. (Exercise is known to stimulate bowel activity.) Increase your consumption of high-fiber foods such as fruits, vegetables, and oat bran. Drink lots of water. I recommend at least four pieces of fruit per day (good choices include oranges and apples), and try to include four servings of vegetables too (good choices are raw carrots, red or green pepper, and broccoli). Finally, set eight glasses of water as your daily goal. If you are eating fruits and vegetables, drinking water, and exercising, you will also be less likely to gain weight.

37. Try a Smoking Cessation Aid

For many people, the tips just outlined are helpful but not sufficient to achieve their goal of a smoke-free life. If you smoke first thing in the morning or more than a pack a day, you may well benefit from a smoking cessation aid. In addition to nicotine replacement (gum, patch, inhaler, and nicotine nasal spray), smokers now have another option: bupropion (also called Wellbutrin or Zyban). This choice may be even more beneficial than the nicotine replacement. Bupropion pills are taken twice a day. They may be used alone or in combination with nicotine replacement.

The nicotine patch is a popular form of nicotine replacement and is currently available without a prescription. There are several different brands, including Habitrol (manufactured by Ciba-Geigy), Nicoderm (Hoechst Marion Roussel, Inc.), Nicotrol (Pharmacia AB), and Prostep (American Cyanamid Company). With the exception of Prostep, which comes in only two doses, each patch comes in three dosing levels. The idea is to gradually reduce your nicotine exposure over a period of eight to sixteen weeks. A very recent article from the Mayo Clinic suggested that people who smoke more than a pack of cigarettes per day might benefit from utilizing two patches initially. (Two patches will provide 42 mg of nicotine over a 24-hour period.) In this case, I would recommend using 42 mg (or two patches) per day for six weeks, followed by 21 mg for up to six weeks, followed by 14 mg per day for six weeks. Finally, end the use of the patch with the 7-mg-per-day dose for up to six weeks.

Instructions on exactly how to use the patch are provided with each package. With the nicotine patch, people break the smoking habit in two steps. First, they get rid of the repetitive hand-to-mouth ritual; then they gradually reduce their dependence on nicotine by slowly withdrawing from it. Studies have shown that the successful quit rate is higher with the patch than quitting cold turkey. In addition, it appears that people who use the patch gain less weight as they quit.

The patch is generally placed on a person's upper shoulder (over the tricep muscle), on the upper part of the chest wall (above the breasts) or the upper part of one's back. Because some people are sensitive to the adhesive in the patch and can develop a skin rash, I recommend placing your patch on the left arm on even days of the month and on the right on odd days. Or you can consider rotating from the right arm to the chest wall to the left arm and then the back. If your skin is sensitive to the patch, or if you want to try an alternate form of nicotine replacement, consider the use of nicotine gum, nicotine nasal spray, or the new Nicotrol inhaler. I find the gum and inhaler especially useful for people who really need to have something in their mouths.

The nicotine gum is available as 2- or 4-mg doses. I think the 4-mg dose provides better relief from withdrawal symptoms than the 2-mg dose. The gum comes with instructions, but a few points are still worth noting since, in my experience, many people use this gum improperly. The gum works by allowing you to absorb nicotine through your gums, so it needs to be in contact with them. After chewing for about 20 seconds or so, park the gum between your cheek and gums, where the nicotine will be easily absorbed and your craving diminished. It is also important to know that eating or drinking while you are chewing the gum, especially drinking carbonated beverages, diminishes your ability to absorb the nicotine.

The nicotine spray has been proven to aid in smoking cessation. There have been three large trials comparing the nicotine spray (marketed by McNeil Consumer Products) with a placebo spray. Table 14 shows the quit rate in the 730 participants of these three studies (369 received the Nicotrol nasal spray and 361 received the placebo):

TABLE 14 Percent of Group Off Cigarettes at:

	6 Wks.	*3 Mos.*	*6 Mos.*	*12 Mos.*
Nicotrol Spray	49–58%	41–45%	31–35%	23–27%
Placebo	21–32%	17–20%	12–15%	10–15%

The usual dose of the Nicotrol nasal spray is two sprays (one in each nostril). I ask my patients not to sniff, swallow, or inhale through the nose as they are spraying. I also ask them to tip the head back slightly as they deliver the spray. The two sprays provide 1 mg of nicotine. After two sprays, blood levels of nicotine rise rapidly. Maximum blood levels are achieved for most people between four and fifteen minutes after a dose. A 1-mg dose allows most people to achieve the same nicotine blood level as after smoking a cigarette. People with a cold or runny nose will take about 30 percent longer to achieve a similar nicotine blood level because of the delay in absorption.

I generally ask my patients to start out with one to two doses per hour, which can be increased up to a maximum recommended daily dose of 40 mg (80 sprays). I also recommend no more than five doses (ten sprays) over the course of an hour. After 10 to 12 weeks of use, I generally recommend tapering the use of the spray. Many people start by cutting their dose to one spray instead of two, and then work on increasing the length of time between sprays.

Based on the results of a study published in the *British Journal of Medicine* in 1999, I now use the spray as a follow-up to the nicotine patch. In this study, titled "Nicotine Nasal Spray With Nicotine Patch for Smoking Cessation: A Randomized Trial With Six-Year Follow-Up," Dr. T. Blondal and colleagues found that people who were treated with a nicotine patch in decreasing dose for five months, followed by a year in which the nicotine spray was available, were twice as likely to stay off cigarettes for six years as compared to people who had five months of the patch followed by the availability of a placebo (no nicotine) spray.

I tell my patients that they can continue to use the nicotine spray for as long as they need it. It has been my experience that many patients will use it once or twice a week for as long as a year or two and that many keep it with them for even longer "just in case." I use the nicotine spray following the nicotine patch, along with the gum, nicotine inhaler, or bupropion. I would not recommend that the spray be used at the same time as the patch, because patients wear the patch continuously.

Are there side effects from the Nicotrol nasal spray? Almost universally people complain of nasal irritation. This improves over time but can be troublesome. Other complaints include runny nose, throat irritation, watering eyes, sneezing, and cough.

The new nicotine inhaler holds promise for people who are not only addicted to cigarettes but also need the repetitive hand-to-mouth ritual. Marketed by McNeil Consumer Products Co., the Nicotrol Inhaler is available by prescription from your doctor. The inhaler consists of a mouthpiece and a plastic cartridge (which is attached to the mouthpiece) capable of delivering 4 mg of nicotine to the mouth and lungs of the user. Ten puffs of the inhaler is roughly the equivalent of one puff on a conventional cigarette. Each cartridge is designed to be used for about 20 minutes of continuous puffing. You may use as many as 20 cartridges per day for about 12 weeks. After this, a gradual reduction in the number of cartridges used per day is recommended. The Nicotrol Inhaler should be used for no longer than six months. Although the Nicotrol Inhaler is typically well tolerated, some people note slight irritation in the mouth and throat.

Recently bupropion (also known as Wellbutrin or Zyban) has been found to be a very effective smoking cessation tool. Bupropion was originally used as an antidepressant. Interest in this medication increased dramatically when it was also found to be useful in helping smokers kick the habit. One small study randomly assigned 42 patients to receive either bupropion or a placebo. At the end of two years, 50 percent of those who were assigned to bupropion remained smoke-free, whereas all of those taking the placebo had resumed smoking.

Because bupropion is a prescription medication, you will be able to decide along with your physician if it is the right choice for you. People with a history of seizures should not take this medication. If you are already on another antidepressant, your doctor may choose to substitute bupropion. This, of course, may not always be appropriate. When we prescribe bupropion, we give our patients the following instructions:

Dose

Begin with 150 milligrams (one pill) once daily in the morning for three days. If you tolerate one pill per day, increase to 150 milligrams twice a day (two pills). Separate the pills by at least eight hours. You should continue to smoke for the first week you are taking bupropion. On day eight, stop smoking. We recommend using bupropion for at least seven to twelve weeks. It is possible that you may require this drug for longer than twelve weeks.

Side Effects

The most common side effects include dry mouth, constipation, headache, and trouble sleeping.

Precautions

As mentioned earlier, you should not take bupropion if you have a history of seizures. Also, if you have been taking a monoamine oxidase inhibitor, you must discontinue this medication at least two weeks prior to beginning bupropion.

It is important to continue smoking for the first week on bupropion. Before you can expect it to help you quit smoking, a certain level of this medication must build up in your bloodstream. This occurs about one week after you begin taking it.

How effective are these medications? In a very recent study published in the *New England Journal of Medicine*, Jorenby and colleagues examined the impact of the bupropion alone, the nicotine patch alone, or the two in combination, as compared to placebo (sugar pill plus an inactive patch) in 893 smokers. All participants received counseling and supportive phone calls throughout the 12-month study. At the end of the study, the quit rate was 5.6 percent in the placebo group, 9.8 percent in the nicotine patch group, 18.4 percent in the bupropion alone group, and 22.5 percent in the combined treatment group. People treated with any form of nicotine replacement (that is, either the patch or bupropion) experienced less weight gain and fewer withdrawal symptoms.

No matter how you do it, quitting smoking is difficult, but you are worth the effort required. Believe in yourself, and just keep trying. If you slip up, rather than chastising yourself and wallowing in guilt (and more cigarettes), learn from the experience. Why did it happen? Try to make certain that you don't put yourself in that particular situation again.

As you become a nonsmoker, you are likely to experience some setbacks along the way. Ultimately, if you continue to try, you will be successful. As a nonsmoker you will be much healthier. Not only will your cholesterol improve, but your risk of lung disease, heart disease, and stroke will decrease dramatically, not to mention your risk of many forms of cancer. You know you want to do it. I know you can.

PART SIX

Medications and Other Treatments

38. Be Open to the Idea of Medications

At some point, your doctor may ask you to begin taking a cholesterol-lowering medication. Some people become terribly upset when this suggestion is made. Patients have told me that they are very concerned about possible side effects (especially the potential impact on the liver). Other people tell me that the idea of going on a medication makes them feel like a failure. On the other hand, I have had a few patients who were delighted at the prospect of beginning a cholesterol-lowering medication. These people feel that being on a medication will allow them to go back to eating whatever they wanted.

In terms of side effects, the most common concern my patients voice is the fear of liver toxicity. The first and most important thing to say is that liver toxicity is very, very rare. However, because it *can* occur with some of the commonly used cholesterol-lowering medications, it is equally important to point out that the liver is one of the few organs in the body that can repair itself. The liver is most effective in repairing itself if the injury is caught quickly. With careful monitoring of liver functions through simple blood tests, it is rare for any cholesterol-lowering medication to cause an irreversible complication.

When a physician initiates cholesterol-lowering medication, he or she obtains a blood test of liver functions (to establish a baseline for comparison). Six to twelve weeks after beginning the medication, the test is repeated. If there is a problem, the physician can stop the medication. As a rule, liver functions return to normal very quickly (within days to a few weeks). If everything looks fine with the first follow-up lab test, your doctor may choose to recheck your liver functions every three to six months. In some cases, it is acceptable to monitor liver functions on a yearly basis.

Many patients ask me what sort of symptoms they might experience if they were having a problem with their liver. The most common symptoms include nausea, fatigue, and abdominal discomfort. Certainly jaundice (yellow discoloration of a person's skin or the whites of his or her eyes) would be a cause for concern, even in the absence of other symptoms.

Being on a cholesterol-lowering medication does not mean you are a failure. Many people have genetic cholesterol abnormalities. Even though diet and exercise will improve the cholesterol levels of such people, they almost universally require medications as well.

If you are a person who has already suffered a heart attack, had an angioplasty, stent placement, or undergone bypass surgery, you will likely also need to take medication to lower your cholesterol. This is because the cholesterol goals for a person with heart disease are much stricter than those for other people. Other groups of people who have the same cholesterol goals as people with heart disease are men and women who have had a stroke, who have diabetes, and who have been told that they have blockages in their leg arteries. The reason these people have the same strict cholesterol goals is that they are also at high risk for developing heart disease.

There are some people who have a genetic disorder called familial hypercholesterolemia who need even more than just diet, exercise, and cholesterol-lowering medications. In our practice, we have a group of people who require a procedure called LDL apheresis. This is a dialysis-like procedure that cleanses the blood of LDL cholesterol and must be performed every two weeks. Our center is one of 34 centers nationwide to offer LDL apheresis. If your cholesterol is still very high despite maximum medications, you may be a candidate for this procedure. LDL apheresis can lower your LDL cholesterol level by as much as 70 percent.

As mentioned earlier, being on medication does not mean that you should abandon your diet or exercise efforts. And if you are taking a supplement that has worked well for you, continuing to take it will likely mean that you'll require a lower dose of medicine. In fact, one study published in the *Journal of the American Medical Association* found that only 50 percent of people taking a cholesterol-lowering drug alone reached their cholesterol goals, whereas 80 percent who followed a diet *and* faithfully took their medication reached their cholesterol goals.

Many people do not realize that cholesterol-lowering medications are a lifelong proposition. Unlike antibiotics, which may require only 10 days of therapy, cholesterol-lowering drugs work only as long as you are taking them. Once discontinued, cholesterol levels will increase.

Taking your medication correctly and faithfully can greatly reduce your risk of having a heart attack or requiring angioplasty or bypass surgery. We used to think that it took a year or two before the benefits of cholesterol-lowering medications could be seen. A number of very recent trials have shown that, in fact, the benefit occurs very quickly. In July of 1999, Dr. Bertram Pitt and colleagues published the dramatic findings of the Atorvastatin Versus Revascularization Treatments (AVERT) study in the *New England Journal of Medicine*. In this study, 341 cardiac patients from 37 different centers were treated with either angioplasty (a procedure in which a thin catheter containing an inflatable balloon is used to open a blocked coronary artery) or high-dose atorvastatin (Lipitor), a cholesterol-lowering medication.

At the end of 18 months, the patients assigned to Lipitor experienced 36 percent fewer cardiac events. The patients who were assigned to the angioplasty arm of this study were actually allowed to receive cholesterol-lowering medications too. The difference in cardiac events really seemed to stem from the fact that although both groups started the study with nearly identical LDL cholesterol levels (145 mg/dl), at the end of 18 months patients who received Lipitor at a dose of 80 mg/day enjoyed an LDL cholesterol level of 77 mg/dl, while patients who were treated with angioplasty had LDL cholesterol levels hovering around 119 mg/dl. Their doctors did put them on a cholesterol-lowering medication, but failed to increase their dose to achieve the LDL cholesterol goal set by the National Cholesterol Education Program (NCEP) of less than 100 mg/dl. I think a better goal is less than 80 mg/dl, and this study is one of the reasons I feel this way.

Even more recently, the Myocardial Ischemia Reduction with Aggressive Cholesterol-Lowering (MIRACL) study was presented at the American Heart Association's national cardiac conference (held in New Orleans in November 2000). Dr. Anders Olsson from Sweden and Gregory Schwartz from the University of Colorado Health Sciences Center presented their findings.

MIRACL included 3,086 patients who were hospitalized because of unstable angina (chest pain or pressure resulting from insufficient blood flow and oxygen delivery to the heart muscle—typically, the result of blockages within the coronary arteries) or heart attack. The study was conducted in 19 countries with 122 medical centers participating. Within 96 hours of hospitalization, patients were treated with either high-dose atorvastatin (Lipitor) and a low-fat diet or a low-fat diet plus a placebo. At the end of only 16 weeks, cardiac events were reduced by a full 16 percent in the Lipitor-treated group. Even more impressive, strokes were reduced by 50 percent in this high-risk population of men and women. These studies certainly suggest that cholesterol-lowering medications can have a dramatic and rapid impact.

Some cholesterol-altering medications—for example, Mevacor, Zocor, Lipitor, Pravachol, and Lescol—lower LDL cholesterol and have a lesser impact on HDL cholesterol and triglycerides. Other medications primarily lower triglycerides and raise HDL cholesterol. These drugs may also lower LDL cholesterol (Tricor and Niaspan are examples) or may have virtually no impact on the LDL cholesterol (Lopid).

While the major benefit of HMG CoA Reductase inhibitors is clearly cholesterol reduction (which dramatically lowers the risk of cardiac events and death), there appear to be interesting additional benefits to these drugs. Preliminary data suggest that this class of drugs may decrease the risk of osteoporosis in women and reduce the risk of developing Alzheimer's disease.

Note: Occasionally, a single cholesterol-lowering medication fails to fully normalize a person's cholesterol levels. In such a situation, physicians will ask a patient to take two medications. Because this increases the risk of possible side effects, people on combination therapy should be seen frequently for monitoring of liver and muscle functions.

In the next few pages, I will list the major medications used in treating cholesterol along with their brand names and generic designations. I will discuss how the medication works, the best way to take it, and the possible side effects. Table 15 briefly lists these medications:

TABLE 15 Cholesterol-Lowering Medications

Class of Drug	Drug Name*	Impact on Cholesterol and Triglycerides		
		LDL	TRIGS**	HDL
Bile Acid Sequestrants	Cholestyramine (Questran)	D	I	I
	Colestipol (Colestid)	D	I	I
	Colesevelam (WelChol)	D	N/I	I
Niacin	Nicotinic acid (Niaspan)	D	D	I
HMG CoA Reductase Inhibitors	Lovastatin (Mevacor)	D	D	I
	Simvastatin (Zocor)	D	D	I

Class of Drug	Drug Name*	Impact on Cholesterol and Triglycerides		
		LDL	TRIGS**	HDL
HMG CoA	Pravastatin	D	D	I
Reductase	(Pravachol)			
Inhibitors	Fluvastatin (Lescol)	D	D	I
(continued)	Atorvastatin (Lipitor)	D	D	I
Fibric Acid	Gemfibrozil (Lopid)	N	D	I
Derivatives	Fenofibrate (Tricor)	D	D	I

* The first drug name given is the generic designation; the one in parentheses
is the brand name.
** Trigs = triglycerides
D = decrease, I = increase, N = neutral

Medications within a class generally have the same impact
on lipids. The exception to this rule is within the fibric acid
derivatives; while Lopid is neutral in terms of LDL, Tricor
has the beneficial impact of lowering this lipoprotein. Within
the class of HMG CoA Reductase inhibitors (also called
statins), there is a broad range of lipid-altering potential.
Although all statins favorably alter LDL and triglycerides,
Lipitor has the greatest LDL and triglyceride-lowering
potential (up to a 55 percent and 45 percent reduction,
respectively). On the other hand, even though all statins
have a positive impact on HDL, Zocor has the most dramatic
impact — especially at high doses.

39. Talk to Your Doctor About Questran

Questran binds bile acids (which are made from cholesterol) within the intestine and excretes them into the stool.

Questran also increases the number of LDL-removing receptors on the liver cell.

Effect

Depending on the dose, Questran can lower the LDL cholesterol by 15 to 20 percent. People who have high triglycerides at baseline may experience an increase in triglycerides while taking Questran. Therefore, Questran is not generally recommended if a person has high triglycerides. HDL generally increases by about 8 to 10 percent while taking Questran.

How to Take It/Dose

The usual starting dose of Questran is one packet or scoopful (four grams) twice a day. Some people may require as much as two packets or scoops three times a day.

Side Effects

The most common complaint is constipation. (In fact, Questran is sometimes used to treat diarrhea.) Constipation can be minimized by slowly increasing the dose of Questran and by increasing daily water intake. Other less common side effects include gas and nausea.

When to Take It

It is best to take this medication just before a meal. However, because Questran can interfere with the absorption of other medications, it is best to take the other medications two hours before or four to six hours after Questran. (This issue of interfering with the absorption of other drugs does not appear to be an issue with WelChol. As a result, WelChol is my first-choice bile-acid sequestrant. See the section on WelChol for more information.)

How to Prepare

1. Dissolve one packet or scoop in four to six ounces of water or juice. Never take it in dry form.
2. Let the mixture stand without stirring for one to two minutes.
3. Stir until it is completely mixed; it will not dissolve. Drink slowly to minimize belching.

Follow-Up

Because the bile-acid sequestrants are not absorbed into the bloodstream (they work in the intestine), they do not cause liver toxicity. It is therefore not necessary to monitor liver functions while on this class of drug.

Other

Because Questran can interfere with the absorption of folic acid and possibly other essential nutrients, I recommend taking a daily multivitamin. Questran is not absorbed into the blood, so there is no risk of liver toxicity.

40. Talk to Your Doctor About Colestid

Colestid binds bile acids (which are made from cholesterol) within the intestine and excretes them into the stool. In addition, Colestid increases the number of LDL-removing receptors on the liver cell.

Effect

Depending on the dose, Colestid can lower the LDL cholesterol by 15 to 20 percent. People who have high triglycerides at baseline may experience an increase while taking Colestid. As such, Colestid is not generally recommended if a person has high triglycerides. HDL generally increases by about 8 to 10 percent while taking Colestid.

How to Take It/Dose

The usual starting dose of Colestid is one packet or scoopful (five grams) twice a day. Some people may require as much as two packets or scoops three times a day.

Side Effects

Patients' most common complaint is constipation. (In fact, Colestid is sometimes used to treat diarrhea.) Constipation can be minimized by slowly increasing the dose of Colestid and by increasing daily water intake. Other less common side effects include gas and nausea.

When to Take It

It is best to take this medication just before a meal. However, because Colestid can interfere with the absorption of other medications, it is best to take the other medications two hours before or four to six hours after Colestid. (This issue of interfering with the absorption of other drugs does not appear to be an issue with WelChol. As a result, WelChol is my first-choice bile-acid sequestrant. See the section on WelChol for more information.)

How to Prepare

1. Dissolve one packet or scoop in four to six ounces of water or juice. Never take it in dry form.

2. Let the mixture stand without stirring for one to two minutes.

3. Stir until it is completely mixed; it will not dissolve. Drink slowly to minimize belching.

Follow-Up

Because the bile-acid sequestrants are not absorbed into the bloodstream (they work in the intestine), they do not cause liver toxicity. It is therefore not necessary to monitor liver functions while on this class of drug.

Other

Because Colestid can interfere with the absorption of folic acid and possibly other essential nutrients, I recommend taking a daily multivitamin. Colestid is not absorbed into the blood, so there is no risk of liver toxicity.

Colestid (Tablets)

Colestid is also available in an easier-to-take tablet form. Each tablet contains a one-gram dose. The usual starting dose is two tablets (two grams) twice a day. Some people may require as many as 16 tablets per day. It is important to drink at least eight ounces of water with each dose.

41. Talk to Your Doctor About WelChol

WelChol binds bile acids (which are made from cholesterol) within the intestine and excretes them into the stool. In addition, WelChol increases the number of LDL-removing receptors on the liver cell.

Effect

Depending on the dose, WelChol can lower the LDL cholesterol by 15 to 20 percent. People who have high triglycerides at baseline may experience an increase while taking WelChol. Therefore, WelChol is not generally recommended if a person has high triglycerides. HDL generally increases by about 8 to 10 percent while taking WelChol.

How to Take It/Dose

The usual starting dose of WelChol is either three tablets (625 mg each) twice a day or six tablets once a day, with food. If a person complains of constipation, I ask him or her to slowly increase to the full dose over a period of a few weeks, rather than beginning a WelChol treatment program with the full dose.

Side Effects

The most common complaint is constipation. Constipation can be minimized by slowly increasing the dose.

When to Take It

It is best to take this medication just before a meal. WelChol does not interfere with the absorption of other drugs, and therefore does not need to be separated in time from other medications. This is a major issue, since many people who are taking WelChol are on several other medications. For this reason, WelChol is my first-choice bile-acid sequestrant.

Follow-Up

Because the bile-acid sequestrants are not absorbed into the bloodstream (they work in the intestine), they do not cause liver toxicity. It is therefore not necessary to monitor liver functions while on this class of drug.

42. Talk to Your Doctor About Niaspan

Although all the actions of niacin are not known, it is clear that Niaspan (a drug that has the vitamin niacin as its active ingredient) lowers the liver's ability to produce very low-density lipoprotein (VLDL). VLDL is a triglyceride-rich lipoprotein produced in the liver. Once it reaches the blood-stream, VLDL is ultimately converted to LDL. Both LDL and VLDL can block the arteries.

Because VLDL is a triglyceride-rich lipoprotein, it is not surprising that triglycerides fall with the use of Niaspan. LDL levels also fall when Niaspan is taken regularly, since there is less VLDL to reach the bloodstream and be converted to LDL. Of all the cholesterol-altering medications currently available, Niaspan is most effective at raising a low HDL level. Although the mechanism by which Niaspan raises HDL is not completely understood, it appears to involve an enzyme called hepatic triglyceride lipase.

Effect

Depending on the dose of Niaspan, LDL can fall by 10 to 20 percent, triglycerides typically drop by 20 to 25 percent, and HDL increases by 20 to 25 percent. Maximum doses of Niaspan have also been shown to lower lipoprotein(a) by as much as 20 percent. Lipoprotein(a) is a genetically predetermined lipoprotein. If a person's lipoprotein(a) level is elevated, diet and exercise will not lower it. The only medications that have been shown to lower lipoprotein(a) are niacin and estrogen.

How to Take It/Dose

Niaspan is a bedtime medication. Following a few simple guidelines minimizes the major side effects, which are flushing and itching of the skin. We start patients on the drug gradually, beginning at 500 mg for four weeks and then increasing them to 1,000 mg. If a 1,000-mg dose does not achieve the desired effect, we increase to a maximum of 2,000 mg per day.

We recommend taking an aspirin about 30 minutes prior to taking the drug. Both the flushing and itching side effects are believed to be caused by the release of prostaglandins. Prostaglandins are a natural substance made by the body. They cause all the little blood vessels on the surface of the skin to dilate. This results in increased blood flow to the skin and hence a warm flushed feeling. Aspirin blocks the release of these prostaglandins.

Because hot beverages, hot showers, and alcohol can all cause flushing on their own, we advise patients to avoid these things within an hour of taking Niaspan.

Finally, taking Niaspan with a small snack (a few crackers, a glass of skim milk, a bowl of cereal, a banana, or a graham cracker) slows its absorption and therefore minimizes the flushing and itching.

Side Effects

The most common side effects, as just noted, are flushing and itching. In general, we ask people to stick it out for two to four weeks. Over this time period, side effects generally diminish greatly or disappear altogether. Occasionally, a patient will complain of nausea with Niaspan. Although this, too, generally goes away with time, if it persists it is crucial to check liver functions via a simple blood test.

When to Take It

As mentioned above, Niaspan should be taken at bedtime. One of the benefits of this is that if you flush, you will flush in your sleep.

Follow-Up

While on Niaspan, it is important to follow up regularly with your doctor. He or she will want to test your liver functions regularly. In some patients, blood-sugar and uric-acid levels should also be checked. All of these are simple blood tests.

Precautions

Niaspan is an excellent medication, but it does have a number of serious potential complications. It can worsen diabetes in some people, although recent studies indicate that many diabetics can do quite well with this drug. It can cause gout in predisposed individuals. Although this is quite rare, liver-function abnormalities can occur. Finally, in a person with a history of peptic-ulcer disease, Niaspan can occasionally increase the risk of a recurrence.

Other

In general, I use only the prescription form of niacin (Niaspan). Niaspan appears to be the only once-a-day form of niacin that does not carry a significant increase in the risk of liver toxicity. Niacin is, however, also available in many over-the-counter preparations that must be taken three times a day. If you use an over-the-counter preparation, please be careful not to purchase slow-release, or "no flush" niacin, as it increases the risk of liver toxicity. If you take an over-the-counter preparation, make sure to discuss this with your physician. The immediate-release over-the-counter preparations should be taken in a dose of 500 mg three times a day; again, this dose should be worked up to gradually. One problem with the immediate-release preparations of niacin is that they need to be taken three times a day (with breakfast, lunch, and supper). Failure to take the immediate-release niacin three times a day can make it almost impossible to get rid of the flushing and itching side effects.

Finally, if you are buying over-the-counter niacin, make sure you do not purchase nicotinamide. While this "cousin" of niacin does not cause flushing or itching, it has no effect on cholesterol.

43. Talk to Your Doctor About Mevacor

Mevacor partially blocks the enzyme HMG CoA Reductase. This enzyme regulates the production of cholesterol in the liver, and in fact, in all the cells within our bodies. The net result of its blockage is a profound reduction in total and LDL cholesterol. A small improvement in triglycerides and HDL is also seen.

Effect

Depending on the dose, Mevacor will lower LDL by 25 to 40 percent. People with elevated triglycerides will see a modest reduction. HDL may increase slightly.

How to Take It/Dose

The usual dose is 10 to 80 mg per day. Mevacor should be taken with the evening meal. At doses over 20 mg, it should be taken twice a day (in other words, a 40-mg dose should be taken as 20 mg twice a day). The best times to take a split dose are at breakfast and dinner. If you miss a dose, take it as soon as you remember. If it is almost time for your next dose, skip the missed dose and go back to your regular schedule. Do not take a double dose.

Side Effects

The side effects of Mevacor are typically mild and don't tend to last. Possible side effects include constipation, diarrhea, abdominal cramps, nausea, headache, and muscle aches.

Follow-Up

While on Mevacor you will need regular follow-up with your physician, who will want to check your liver functions periodically.

Precautions

If you develop fever, muscle cramping, and weakness while on Mevacor, you may have developed a rare complication called myositis. Of course, these symptoms may just be the flu. In such a case, your doctor will do a simple blood test to check your blood level of muscle enzymes. If you have a significantly elevated level of muscle enzymes, Mevacor will be discontinued.

44. Talk to Your Doctor About Zocor

Zocor partially blocks the enzyme HMG CoA Reductase. This enzyme regulates the production of cholesterol in the liver, and in fact, in all the cells within our bodies. The net result of this blockage is a profound reduction in total and LDL cholesterol. A small improvement in triglycerides and HDL is also seen.

Effect

Depending on the dose, Zocor will lower LDL by 25 to 45 percent. In people with elevated triglycerides, a modest reduction can be seen. HDL may increase. Of all the available drugs in this class, Zocor appears to have the greatest impact on HDL.

How to Take It/Dose

Zocor should be taken at bedtime. The usual dose is 5 to 80 mg per day. If you miss a dose, take it as soon as you remember. If it is almost time for your next dose, skip the missed dose and go back to your regular schedule. Do not take a double dose.

Side Effects

The side effects of Zocor are typically mild and don't tend to last. Possible side effects include constipation, diarrhea, abdominal cramps, nausea, headache, and muscle aches.

Follow-Up

While on Zocor, you will need regular follow-up with your physician, who will want to periodically check your liver functions.

Precautions

If you develop fever, muscle cramping, and weakness while on Zocor, you may have developed a rare complication called myositis. Of course, these symptoms may just be the flu. In such a case, your doctor will do a simple blood test to check your blood level of muscle enzymes. If you have a significantly elevated level of muscle enzymes, Zocor will be discontinued.

45. Talk to Your Doctor About Pravachol

Pravachol partially blocks the enzyme HMG CoA Reductase. This enzyme regulates the production of cholesterol in the liver, and in fact, in all the cells within our bodies. The net result of this blockage is a profound reduction in total and LDL cholesterol. A small improvement in triglycerides and HDL is also seen.

Effect

Depending on the dose, Pravachol will lower LDL by 20 to 32 percent. In people with elevated triglycerides, a modest reduction can be seen. HDL may also increase slightly.

How to Take It/Dose

Pravachol should be taken at bedtime. The usual dose is 10 to 40 mg per day. If you miss a dose, take it as soon as you remember. If it is almost time for your next dose, skip the missed dose and go back to your regular schedule. Do not take a double dose.

Side Effects

The side effects of Pravachol are typically mild and don't tend to last. Possible side effects include constipation, diarrhea, abdominal cramps, nausea, headache, and muscle aches.

Follow-Up

While on Pravachol you will need regular follow-up with your physician, who will want to periodically check your liver functions.

Precautions

If you develop fever, muscle cramping, and weakness while on Pravachol, you may have developed a rare complication called myositis. Of course, these symptoms may just be the flu. In such a case, your doctor will do a simple blood test to check your blood level of muscle enzymes. If you have a significantly elevated level of muscle enzymes, Pravachol will be discontinued.

46. Talk to Your Doctor About Lescol

Lescol partially blocks the enzyme HMG CoA Reductase. This enzyme regulates the production of cholesterol in the liver, and in fact, in all the cells within our bodies. The net result of this blockage is a profound reduction in total and LDL cholesterol. A small improvement in triglycerides and HDL is also seen.

Effect

Depending on the dose, Lescol will lower LDL by 20 to 35 percent. In people with elevated triglycerides, a modest reduction can be seen. HDL may also increase slightly.

How to Take It/Dose

Lescol should be taken at bedtime. The usual dose is 20 to 80 mg per day. If you miss a dose, take it as soon as you remember. If it is almost time for your next dose, skip the missed dose and go back to your regular schedule. Do not take a double dose.

Side Effects

The side effects of Lescol are typically mild and don't tend to last. Possible side effects include constipation, diarrhea, abdominal cramps, nausea, headache, and muscle aches.

Follow-Up

While on Lescol you will need regular follow-up with your physician, who will want to periodically check your liver functions.

Precautions

If you develop fever, muscle cramping, and weakness while on Lescol, you may have developed a rare complication called myositis. Of course, these symptoms may just be the flu. In such a case, your doctor will do a simple blood test to check your blood level of muscle enzymes. If you have a significantly elevated level of muscle enzymes, Lescol will be discontinued.

Note

A new extended-release preparation of Lescol (Lescol XL 80 mg) has just become available. This preparation appears to lower LDL much more substantially, on the order of 33 to 35 percent.

47. Talk to Your Doctor About Lipitor

Lipitor partially blocks the enzyme HMG CoA Reductase. This enzyme regulates the production of cholesterol in the liver and in fact, in all the cells within our bodies. The net result of this blockage is a profound reduction in total and LDL cholesterol. A small improvement in triglycerides and HDL is also seen.

Effect

Depending on the dose, Lipitor will lower LDL by 33 to 55 percent. In people with elevated triglycerides, a substantial reduction can be seen. HDL may increase slightly.

How to Take It/Dose

One benefit of Lipitor is that it is the only drug in the "statin" family which can be taken anytime, day or night, with or without food. The usual dose is 10 to 80 mg per day.

If you miss a dose, take it as soon as you remember. If it is almost time for your next dose, skip the missed dose and go back to your regular schedule. Do not take a double dose.

Side Effects

The side effects of Lipitor are typically mild and don't tend to last. Possible side effects include constipation, diarrhea, abdominal cramps, nausea, headache, and muscle aches.

Follow-Up

While on Lipitor you will need regular follow-up with your physician, who will want to periodically check your liver functions.

Precautions

If you develop fever, muscle cramping, and weakness while on Lipitor, you may have developed a rare complication called myositis. Of course, these symptoms may just be the flu. In such a case, your doctor will do a simple blood test to check your blood level of muscle enzymes. If you have a significantly elevated level of muscle enzymes, Lipitor will be discontinued.

48. Talk to Your Doctor About Lopid

Lopid increases the activity of lipoprotein lipase, the enzyme responsible for breaking down particles of triglyceride, and increases the amount of cholesterol excreted into the bile. Lopid also appears to slow the production of triglycerides within the liver cells.

Effect

At the standard dose of 600 mg twice a day, Lopid will lower triglycerides by between 25 and 35 percent. HDL cholesterol can be expected to increase by 7 to 20 percent. (Patients with the highest triglyceride levels generally have the greatest increase in HDL.)

How to Take It/Dose

The usual dose is 600 mg twice a day. In very small people (under 100 pounds), we sometimes use 300 mg twice a day. Likewise, people with kidney diseases may require a dose reduction. We generally ask people to take Lopid half an hour before breakfast and half an hour before dinner.

Side Effects

Although most people tolerate Lopid very well, the following side effects have occasionally been reported: nausea, diarrhea, abdominal cramping, dizziness, blurred vision, skin rash, and muscle aches.

Follow-Up

While you are on Lopid, your doctor will want to check your liver functions and periodically run a complete blood count.

Precautions

It is possible that prolonged therapy with Lopid may increase your risk of developing gallbladder disease. If you are taking blood thinners (for example, warfarin or Coumadin), your doctor will want to monitor your prothrombin time (PT) or International Normalized Ratio (INR) closely when you begin Lopid therapy. It is possible that your dose of warfarin may be reduced slightly while on Lopid.

49. Talk to Your Doctor About Tricor

Tricor increases the activity of lipoprotein lipase, the enzyme responsible for breaking down triglyceride-rich particles, and increases the amount of cholesterol excreted into the bile. Tricor also reduces the production of apoprotein C III (an apoprotein which inhibits lipoprotein lipase).

Effect

The ability of Tricor to lower triglycerides, lower LDL, and raise HDL depends on a person's baseline lipid levels. In people with elevated triglyceride levels, the standard dose of 160 mg per day will lower triglycerides between 45 and 55 percent. HDL cholesterol can be expected to increase by about 20 percent. In patients who have an elevated LDL cholesterol level but normal or near-normal triglycerides at baseline, Tricor has been found to lower LDL by 20 to 30 percent. In these patients, triglyceride levels fell more modestly (by about 25 to 30 percent). HDL levels rose in these patients by 10 to 15 percent.

How to Take It/Dose

Tricor should be taken with a meal. Although Tricor is typically prescribed as a single 160-mg tablet per day, this medication is also available as a 54-mg tablet. Some people require only a 54-mg tablet to correct their triglyceride problem. Patients with significant kidney problems should take a reduced dose of Tricor.

Side Effects

Although most people tolerate Tricor very well, the following side effects have occasionally been reported: nausea, abdominal cramping, dizziness, blurred vision, skin rash, and muscle aches.

Follow-Up

While you are on Tricor, your doctor will want to check your liver functions and periodically run a complete blood count.

Precautions

It is possible that prolonged therapy with Tricor may increase your risk of developing gallbladder disease. If you are taking blood thinners (for example, warfarin or Coumadin), your doctor will want to monitor your prothrombin time (PT) or International Normalized Ratio (INR) closely when you begin Tricor therapy. It is possible that your dose of warfarin may be reduced slightly while on Tricor.

50. Don't Give Up Hope — Learn About Medical Procedures and New Drugs

Although most people successfully normalize their LDL cholesterol or triglyceride levels with currently available medications, some people, especially those with genetic cholesterol abnormalities, may not be so lucky. And HDL cholesterol is another situation altogether. Currently available medications *may* help people with very low HDL, but more often they fail to fully correct the low level of this lipoprotein. If this has been your experience, do not give up hope. The future is full of promise. Markedly improved medications and treatments continue to be developed.

In this chapter I will review the genetics of two common cholesterol disorders: familial hypercholesterolemia (FH) and familial combined hyperlipidemia (FCH). FH always leads to markedly elevated LDL cholesterol levels (levels between 250 and 500 mg/dl are not uncommon), and FCH can lead to elevations in either LDL cholesterol or triglycerides (and often, both are elevated). LDL cholesterol can be well over 200 mg/dl and triglycerides can at times be above 1000 mg/dl. People with these disorders may require heroic measures, such as LDL apheresis. They are also likely to be the ones who benefit most from a new group of medications called "superstatins," which I will discuss in detail. This chapter ends with a review of genetic HDL abnormalities and a look at the promising developments in medications and therapies to treat these very serious cholesterol abnormalities.

In my practice, I have a large population of patients with genetic disorders that lead to high LDL cholesterol. As noted earlier, two of the most common are familial hypercholesterolemia (FH) and familial combined hyperlipidemia (FCH). Everyone with FH will have a markedly elevated LDL. The same is true for many (but not all) people with FCH. FH occurs in one in five hundred persons, and FCH develops in one out of a hundred in the general population. (Often people with FCH do not show symptoms of the disorder until they are in their thirties.) FH tends to occur more frequently in certain populations; French Canadians, Afrikaaners in South Africa, the Finnish, the Lebanese, and Ashkenazi Jews all run a much higher risk of this genetic disease. Where I work, in Manchester, New Hampshire, approximately one in one hundred and fifty French Canadians has FH.

FH causes very high cholesterol levels. FH should be suspected in adults when total cholesterol is 340 mg/dl or higher, and in children when total cholesterol is 270 mg/dl. The condition greatly increases one's chances of having an early heart attack, even as early as age 20. Most men with untreated FH will have at least one heart attack by age 55, and most women with this disorder will have the same experience by age 65. Scientists speculate that the reason women with FH have a 10-year advantage is the presence of estrogen. Once a woman with FH goes through menopause, her risk increases rapidly.

FH is caused by an abnormality of the LDL receptor gene. This gene is found on chromosome number 19. People who have inherited a single copy of the abnormal gene have cholesterol levels in the range noted above. A person unfortunate enough to inherit two copies of the abnormal gene often will have a total cholesterol level of over 700 mg/dl. Fortunately, inheriting two copies of the FH gene is extremely rare (one in a million). A person who has a single copy of the FH gene has a 50 percent chance of passing this gene on to his or her children. Once FH is suspected, all first-degree relatives of the person with FH should also be screened. As a rule, 50 percent of those relatives will be found to have FH as well.

People with FH will often have striking findings on physical examination. It is not uncommon to find visible cholesterol deposits (called xanthomas) in the tendons of the hands and feet. Corneal arcus, a deposit of cholesterol that surrounds the colored part of a person's eye, is another sign.

Familial combined hyperlipidemia (FCH) is believed to be the most commonly inherited disorder of cholesterol metabolism. This disorder was first discovered almost 30 years ago by Drs. Joseph Goldstein, Helmut Schrott, William Hazzard, Edward Bierman, and Arno Motulsky, all researchers at the University of Washington. Despite the length of time we have known about FCH, the genetics of this disorder are not well-known. Nonetheless, it is clear that that persons with FCH have a high risk of developing premature heart disease, often suffering their first heart attack before the age of 55.

The words "familial combined hyperlipidemia" refer to what is found on the lipid profiles of affected individuals. An FCH patient can have a lipid profile that reveals a high LDL cholesterol level, a high triglyceride level, or both. A family with FCH can exhibit all these abnormalities. So it is possible that if you have FCH and your sister does too, you may have only an elevated triglyceride level, whereas your sister may have both elevated LDL cholesterol and triglyceride levels.

No matter what your genetic cholesterol abnormality is, it is important to follow the diet and exercise advice outlined in this book. It is fair to say that most people with these disorders will also require cholesterol-lowering medication. And in most cases, a single medication is not sufficient to normalize the cholesterol levels.

There are certainly people with very difficult-to-treat cholesterol in whom double and even triple drug therapy fails to normalize their cholesterol profile. And there will always be those who have difficulty tolerating more than a single medication (due to side effects). In the past, there was little to offer these people. Many experienced unnecessary cardiac events (heart attacks, bypasses, angioplasties) or even died because of their heart disease.

I am happy to say that I am now able to offer my patients a variety of very impressive LDL-cholesterol-lowering options. One option that's approved by the Food and Drug Administration (FDA) is LDL apheresis. LDL apheresis can be thought of as a dialysis for LDL cholesterol. It is a procedure in which blood is removed from the body (via a needle in an arm vein). Once outside the body, the blood is separated into plasma (the liquid in which LDL cholesterol resides) and blood cells. The plasma is then run through a special dextran sulfate cellulose adsorption column. The LDL cholesterol sticks to the adsorption column. Ultimately the LDL-cholesterol–free plasma is reunited with the blood cells when they reenter the body (via a needle into the opposite arm). While outside the body, the blood is treated with heparin to prevent clotting.

LDL apheresis has the ability to lower LDL cholesterol by as much as 70 to 80 percent. The only major drawbacks are the expense of the procedure (it is covered by most insurance plans, however) and the time commitment that's required. Although LDL apheresis can markedly reduce your cholesterol level, it will unfortunately rebound quickly.

Remember, cholesterol is normally manufactured by the body. People who have a genetic cholesterol abnormality will continue to produce cholesterol at a rapid pace following an LDL apheresis procedure. In general, LDL apheresis is repeated every two weeks. Until good gene therapy becomes a reality, we tell our patients that LDL apheresis should be thought of as a lifelong proposition. The entire procedure takes between two and three hours (most people watch a video while it is taking place) and costs anywhere from $2,500 to $3,000. Lest you think your doctor and the nursing staff are getting rich on LDL apheresis, I can tell you that in our clinic all but about $125 goes to pay for the machine and disposables (such as special plastic tubing) used during each procedure. In our clinic, we have a large number of people receiving this therapy.

Kelly is a nine-year-old girl who had a total cholesterol of over 700 mg/dl and an LDL cholesterol of 650 mg/dl when we met her. Unfortunately, she inherited two genes for the development of FH. Unlike patients who have inherited a single gene for FH, people who have inherited two genes typically fail to benefit at all from standard drug therapy. Although Kelly experienced no fall with the statin medications, she did drop her LDL cholesterol by 14 percent with the use of Benecol margarine. Because a 14 percent fall was clearly not sufficient, we knew we had to do something heroic if we were to prevent Kelly from having a heart attack in her teens. Kelly now comes to our center once a week to undergo LDL apheresis.

Before she began the procedure, she had unsightly cholesterol deposits on her face, knees, hands, and ankles. These have literally melted away. From Kelly's point of view, this is the best aspect of the procedure. She explained that the kids in her class made fun of her because of the cholesterol deposits, and when they went away it was easier for her to make friends.

From my point of view, the fact that Kelly's total cholesterol now fluctuates between 100 mg/dl (just after the procedure) and 350 mg/dl (just prior to the procedure) is the most important aspect of her therapy. And while a cholesterol of 350 mg/dl is certainly not normal, it is a whole lot better than it was prior to her therapy. We recently sent Kelly to Children's Hospital in Boston for a stress test, which she passed with flying colors. We were delighted with this result, and bought her a new scooter and helmet to celebrate.

It isn't just people who have inherited two genes for FH who can benefit from LDL apheresis. When Jim was 23 years old, he went to the emergency room complaining of severe chest pain. Luckily, he encountered an excellent physician who didn't look at Jim's age and decide that he couldn't possibly have heart disease. Instead, the doctor took a family history and found that Jim's mother had died at the age of 30 from a heart attack. He also learned that Jim smoked two packs of cigarettes a day. When Jim's LDL cholesterol was tested at 350 mg/dl, the doctor told Jim that he was going to need to stay in the hospital.

Luckily, Jim didn't have a heart attack. But when he failed his stress test the next morning, he found himself in the cardiac catheterization laboratory. This is a procedure in which dye is injected into the coronary arteries via a flexible catheter (a thin, hollow plastic tube) to determine if the arteries have significant blockages.

Unfortunately, Jim was found to have several cholesterol deposits. One required angioplasty, a procedure in which a thin catheter containing an inflatable balloon is used to open a blocked artery. In Jim's case, the angioplasty also involved the placement of a stent, which is a spring much like those found inside a pen. The stent helps prevent the artery from closing again.

Following his hospitalization, Jim gave up smoking, developed a regular exercise program, and followed a low-fat diet. His cardiologist started him first on Zocor and then on Lipitor. Although these drugs managed to drop his LDL from 350 mg/dl to 214 mg/dl, this was still not good enough. (Remember that the goal for LDL cholesterol in a person with heart disease is less than 100 mg/dl.) Jim's doctor added Niaspan, which improved his HDL cholesterol but did little for his LDL cholesterol. His doctor also tried Questran powder, but Jim discontinued it due to bloating. He probably would have done better with the new bile-acid resin called WelChol, but by the time Jim finished with the Questran he refused to try any other bile-acid resin.

At this point, he was referred to me. Considering the many options that had already been tried, it was pretty clear to me that Jim needed LDL apheresis. We cautioned him that he needed to stick with his Lipitor, diet, and exercise program. Jim comes in, movie in hand, every two weeks for his treatment. His most recent pre- and post-treatment lipid values are as follows:

Before LDL Apheresis

Jim's Level	Desirable Level
Total cholesterol 235 mg/dl	< 150 mg/dl
Triglycerides 100 mg/dl	< 100 mg/dl
LDL cholesterol 180 mg/dl	< 100 mg/dl
HDL cholesterol 35 mg/dl	> 45 mg/dl

After LDL Apheresis

Jim's Level	Desirable Level
Total cholesterol 99 mg/dl	< 150 mg/dl
Triglycerides 64 mg/dl	< 100 mg/dl
LDL cholesterol 49 mg/dl	< 100 mg/dl
HDL cholesterol 37 mg/dl	> 45 mg/dl

Not everyone who needs LDL apheresis receives it. Currently only about 35 centers in the country offer this procedure. In addition, some people are unwilling to spend two to three hours every two weeks undergoing this procedure—even if they need it.

Catherine, one of my favorite patients, refused LDL apheresis. When I met her, she had already undergone a carotid endarterectomy, a procedure done to open a carotid (neck) artery that is clogged with cholesterol. A carotid endarterectomy is performed to prevent a stroke from occurring. Her initial cholesterol profile looked like this:

Catherine's Level	Desirable Level
Total cholesterol 363 mg/dl	< 150 mg/dl
Triglycerides 139 mg/dl	< 100 mg/dl
LDL cholesterol 298 mg/dl	< 100 mg/dl
HDL cholesterol 37 mg/dl	> 45 mg/dl

At the time of her referral, she was taking Lopid (600 mg twice a day), Colestid powder (one scoop per day), and Niaspan (1,000 mg per day). She was also taking estrogen, which can lower LDL and raise HDL—but also has a tendency to raise triglycerides.

When we met Catherine, she weighed 148 pounds (she is 64 inches tall). Although her diet was excellent, her portions were too big. We felt she would benefit from weight loss. After working with Mary Card, our registered dietitian, and developing a regular exercise program, Catherine dropped her weight to 132 pounds.

Ultimately, Catherine was following a excellent diet and exercise program, and she was taking Lipitor (at a dose of 80 mg/day), Lopid (600 mg twice a day), Colestid tablets (five grams per day, which was the maximum dose she could tolerate), and estrogen. On this regime, her profile looked like this:

Catherine's Level	**Desirable Level**
Total cholesterol 249 mg/dl	< 150 mg/dl
Triglycerides 79 mg/dl	< 100 mg/dl
LDL cholesterol 193 mg/dl	< 100 mg/dl
HDL cholesterol 41 mg/dl	> 45 mg/dl

For two years, I begged Catherine to consider LDL apheresis. She refused, mainly because she lived 60 minutes from our LDL apheresis center and didn't want to commit to the trip year-round. (In New Hampshire we get snow for at least four months of the year.) But when she ended up having a coronary artery bypass procedure, she changed her mind.

Almost simultaneously, however, I was asked by Astra Zeneca to participate in a clinical trial with a brand new cholesterol-lowering medication called—at that time— ZD4522, or rosuvastatin. This drug is likely to come on the market in July 2002, and will be called Crestor. Crestor is a "superstatin." It is in the same family as other statins, such as Zocor and Lipitor, but appears to be able to lower LDL cholesterol more dramatically. It appears to be just as safe as the currently available statins and has the same side effects. I gave Catherine the option of trying this new medication, with the understanding that if it didn't work we would go forward with the LDL apheresis.

Six weeks after beginning Crestor at 80 mg per day, these were Catherine's cholesterol levels:

Catherine's Level	**Desirable Level**
Total cholesterol 179 mg/dl	< 150 mg/dl
Triglycerides 132 mg/dl	< 100 mg/dl
LDL cholesterol 113 mg/dl	< 100 mg/dl
HDL cholesterol 40 mg/dl	> 45 mg/dl

You might note that Catherine's triglycerides increased slightly; I don't believe this has anything to do with the Crestor. If I tell you these lab studies were drawn on November 29th, I bet you can guess why (hint—it involves a big bird). We currently have 35 patients taking Crestor, and our experience has been overwhelmingly positive. Although 35 patients allows one to get a feel for how a drug is going to perform, it is always wise to reserve judgment until large numbers of people have been treated.

The evidence is beginning to mount on behalf of Crestor. In March of 2001, five clinical trials of Crestor, which included almost 1,700 patients, were presented at the American College of Cardiology meeting in Orlando, Florida. The results of these studies were overwhelmingly positive. Low-dose (5 and 10 mg) Crestor can be expected to lower LDL cholesterol by about 41 and 47 percent, respectively. High-dose Crestor (40 and 80 mg) can be anticipated to lower LDL by as much as 55 and 65 percent, respectively. Crestor also lowers triglycerides by up to 19 percent. While the impact on HDL cholesterol was a little more variable, an increase of 7 to 15 percent should be expected.

Crestor is not the only superstatin currently in clinical trials. Sankyo is beginning trials on a drug currently called NK-104. This drug also promises to dramatically lower LDL cholesterol.

Sometimes combination therapy can do as well as one of the superstatins. In a joint venture, Schering-Plough and Merck have developed a new drug called Ezetimbe. This agent is a selective cholesterol absorption inhibitor (meaning that it works by preventing the absorption of cholesterol from the intestines). A 10-mg dose of Ezetimbe has been shown to lower LDL cholesterol levels by about 20 percent.

While this is not dramatic on its own, when combined with Zocor, Mevacor, and Lipitor the impact has been much more dramatic. A number of studies have been performed. One, combining 10 mg of Ezetimbe with 10 mg of Zocor, yielded a 52 percent reduction in LDL. When 20 mg Zocor was combined with 20 mg Ezetimbe, study subjects enjoyed a 59 percent reduction in their LDL cholesterol. Mevacor at 40 mg in combination with 10 mg of Ezetimbe resulted in an impressive 56 percent reduction in LDL cholesterol. Finally, a small trial combining 10 mg Lipitor with 10 mg Ezetimbe resulted in an LDL cholesterol drop of 56 percent.

None of these trials combined Ezetimbe with high doses of Zocor, Mevacor, or Lipitor. It is very likely that these trials will be performed. Because Ezetimbe appears to be an extremely safe medication, these combinations have the potential to lower LDL by 65 to 70 percent. In the future, Ezetimbe may also be combined with one of the super-statins. These drugs work by different mechanisms, so one could speculate that such a combination might result in as much as an 80 percent reduction in LDL.

Kos Pharmaceuticals is also developing a combination medication, currently called Advicor. Although the Kos combination involves two medications currently available by prescription (lovastatin, or Mevacor; and Niaspan), the Food and Drug Administration still considers this a new drug and requires that clinical trials be performed. Thus far the combination of lovastatin and Niaspan has not produced any surprising side effects (that is, side effects not previously caused by one or the other of the two drugs) and has been very well tolerated. Kos anticipates up to a 45 percent reduction in LDL cholesterol, a 38 percent reduction in triglycerides, and a 29 percent increase in HDL. These reductions were obtained when 2,000 mg of Niaspan were combined with 40 mg of lovastatin. Remember, Niaspan also lowers lipoprotein(a), which has been shown to be a contributing factor in heart disease. Look for Advicor in late 2001 or early 2002.

When it comes to triglycerides, we currently have only two classes of medications: the fibric acid derivatives (Lopid and Tricor) and niacin (Niaspan). I do not know of any new triglyceride medications on the horizon, although all statins have some triglyceride-lowering potential. The superstatins appear to lower triglycerides by as much as 19 percent — probably more in people with high baseline triglycerides. Other fibric acid derivatives are available in Europe and may possibly become available in the United States in the future. These include bezafibrate and ciprofirate.

If your problem is a low HDL cholesterol, you should know that there is likely to be an explosion of new therapies in the next five years. Although HDL cholesterol levels can at times be dramatically improved by either niacin (Niaspan) or the fibric acid derivatives (Lopid or Tricor), this is not always the case. In part, our inability to effectively increase HDL cholesterol levels stems from our lack of a complete understanding of HDL metabolism. Fortunately, over the past few years this understanding has improved dramatically.

In 1996, the first HDL receptor, which is found primarily on liver cells, was identified (by Drs. Susan Acton, Monty Krieger, and colleagues at the Massachusetts Institute of Technology (MIT) in conjunction with Drs. Helen Hobbs and Katherine Landschultz from the University of

Texas Southwestern Medical Center). This receptor, called the class B scavenger receptor or SR-BI, allows cholesterol from HDL to be "dropped off" at the liver, where it can be incorporated into bile acids and passed out into the intestines, where it ultimately ends up in the feces.

In August of 1999 an even more dramatic discovery occurred. Drs. Angela Brooks-Wilson, Michael Hayden, and colleagues from Vancouver, British Columbia, discovered the ABC1 gene and identified its role in HDL metabolism. Dr. Brooks-Wilson and her colleagues were able to learn what the ABC1 gene does by studying people who have defects in this gene.

Tangier disease was first diagnosed by Dr. Donald Fredrickson, who was working at the National Institutes of Health when a five-year-old boy from Tangier Island, Virginia, arrived in his clinic. This little boy had orange tonsils (caused by cholesterol buildup within the tonsils), neurologic problems in his hands and feet (also caused by cholesterol buildup), and an undetectable HDL level. The boy's parents both had low levels of HDL (in the 20 to 25 mg/dl range).

Dr. Fredrickson determined that this was a recessive disorder. (Each parent had a single gene for the disease but did not manifest the disease itself because they had one normal gene; the little boy had received an abnormal gene from each parent and therefore manifested Tangier disease.)

Tangier Island was a "setup" for these recessive diseases. This little island, which is in the middle of the Chesapeake Bay, was settled in the 1680s by a small group of Englishmen and their families. Very few people ever moved off or onto the island. As a result, almost all of the current inhabitants of this island have one of the four surnames of the original settlers. It would stand to reason that given this small gene pool, some genetic disorders might surface.

Although there was little doubt that Tangier disease was a genetic disorder, the precise genetic mutation remained elusive until Dr. Brooks-Wilson and her colleagues identified a defect in the ABC1 gene as the cause of Tangier disease.

What Dr. Brooks-Wilson discovered was that without a properly functioning ABC1 gene, cholesterol cannot get out of a cell. This leads to cholesterol buildup, and if the buildup occurs within the cells lining the heart arteries, the risk of heart disease skyrockets.

In the normal situation when a person has properly functioning ABC1 genes, cholesterol is removed from the cells (for example, cells lining the artery walls) and attaches itself to small disc-shaped particles in our bloodstream. The cholesterol becomes internalized, and the small disc becomes a mature HDL particle. The mature HDL particle brings the cholesterol to the liver for eventual removal from the body. This whole process is known as reverse cholesterol transport.

As you can see, without a properly functioning ABC1 gene, cholesterol stays in the cells, HDL never forms, reverse cholesterol transport never gets "off the starting block," and cardiac risk increases dramatically. People with Tangier disease have two abnormal ABC1 genes and, as noted, are at high risk for cardiac disease. It is also known that simply having one abnormal ABC1 gene (like the parents of the five-year-old boy) results in an increase in cardiac risk.

Although Tangier disease is very rare, having been diagnosed in only about 40 people worldwide, subtle defects in the ABC1 gene are probably quite common. If you have an HDL cholesterol level in the 20 to 25 mg/dl range, you may have some abnormality in your ABC1 gene.

There are now a number of biotech companies actively studying medications designed to upregulate the ABC1 gene. The term "upregulate" is jargon for "make it work harder." Among the companies to watch are CV Therapeutics, in collaboration with Incyte Genomics and the University of Washington. Another company involved in this area is Hyseq, in collaboration with the University of California at San Francisco. Aventis and Merck are two other large companies reported to be actively pursuing work on drugs that will upregulate the ABC1 gene. This research is extremely important, and there is little doubt in my mind that within the next five to six years we will have drugs to help people who have either subtle or major defects in the ABC1 gene.

Not every HDL abnormality can be attributed to problems with the ABC1 gene, however. HDL metabolism is fairly complex; it is possible for your ABC1 gene to be functioning perfectly even though your HDL numbers are too low. Once the HDL cholesterol particle is formed, it can (as mentioned earlier) deliver cholesterol to the liver, or it can send cholesterol to other lipid particles in the bloodstream. These other particles become more cholesterol-rich and ultimately become LDL particles. The LDL particles also travel to the liver to deliver cholesterol.

But not all LDL particles do what they are supposed to do (drop cholesterol off at the liver). Some LDL particles can become chemically modified, or oxidized. These particles are no longer attracted to the liver. Instead, they "drop" their cholesterol off in the artery wall. This occurs in people with high levels of LDL cholesterol, in smokers, and in diabetics. HDL, on the other hand, does not become chemically modified or oxidized.

When the HDL particle delivers cholesterol to the liver directly, it must interact with a receptor on the surface of the liver cells. In order for the HDL to be able to "drop off" its cholesterol, the HDL particle has to be the right match to the receptor. You can think of this as a lock and key. The HDL might have lots of cholesterol to drop off, but if the receptor (or lock) is defective, the key won't work.

As mentioned in the beginning of our HDL discussion, Dr. Susan Acton's group at MIT discovered the class B scavenger receptor, or SR-BI. The SR-BI is the HDL receptor. Some groups are looking at the SR-BI as a target for altering HDL metabolism in the hope of reducing cardiovascular disease.

As noted earlier, the HDL particle sometimes interacts with other lipid particles, giving them the cholesterol to deal with. In order for the HDL particle to "donate" its cholesterol to another lipid particle, a chaperone is necessary. The chaperone is a protein called Cholesterol Ester Transfer Protein (CETP).

In Japan, there are a number of families who have defects in CETP. The result is very high HDL cholesterol levels, and a very low risk of cardiac disease. For a number of reasons, researchers believe that if CETP could intentionally be made defective, HDL levels would increase, and perhaps cardiac risk would decrease. Two companies (Avant Immunotherapeutics and Pfizer) are actively developing CETP inhibitors. In very preliminary studies, Pfizer has found that its agent (CP-529,414) can raise HDL by as much as 70 percent.

Raising HDL does not necessarily mean that cardiac risk will fall. In fact, a few Japanese people with defective CETP and very high HDL levels have suffered from cardiac disease. Nonetheless, CETP inhibitors appear promising.

It may be possible to impact HDL and reverse cholesterol transport without necessarily increasing HDL levels. Esperion Therapeutics is a biopharmaceutical company focused on discovering and developing HDL-targeted therapies. In November 2000, Esperion completed Phase I of their Large Unilamellar Vesicles (LUV) clinical trial program. This same company is also involved in a Phase I Apo A-I Milano (AIM) clinical trial program. Phase I clinical trials are typically very small trials designed to ensure the overall safety of a drug. The drug is generally given to a small number of healthy volunteers.

In the LUV Phase I trial, healthy volunteers were given single and multiple doses of LUV. LUVs are spherical particles made from lipids that can recirculate through the arteries and remove cholesterol from circulation and from the cells in the artery wall. LUVs then transport this cholesterol to the liver.

If LUVs can remove cholesterol from the arteries, especially the heart arteries, they might reverse heart disease — even without HDL levels being increased.

The AIM clinical trial involves an intravenous injection of AIM, which is a variant of Apo A-I (a major component of normal HDL). Apo A-I Milano is present in a small group of people in Northern Italy. These people paradoxically have very low HDL levels, but do not develop coronary disease. It is hoped that AIM will protect against vascular disease by extracting cholesterol from the artery wall and transporting it to the liver for removal. In the phase I trial, Apo A-I Milano appeared to mimic HDL function.

Phase II trials of each of these agents are now getting underway. There is no doubt that the next few years will bring new and exciting therapies for people with low HDL levels.

Throughout this discussion, I have stressed HDL's role in reverse cholesterol transport. Although this is probably HDL's most important role, it is unlikely to be the only way that HDL protects us from cardiovascular disease.

HDL is known to have some potent antioxidant effects. In the context of cardiovascular disease, the role of an antioxidant is to prevent LDL cholesterol from becoming oxidized. Oxidation is a chemical process that occurs within the circulation. When LDL becomes oxidized, it has an easy time getting into the artery wall, where it sets up shop and contributes to the development of atherosclerosis. In order for LDL to get into the artery wall, it must attach itself to the endothelial cells that line the artery. The easiest way for LDL to do this is to attach to something called an adhesion molecule. HDL seems to prevent these adhesion molecules from occurring on the endothelial cells. This again creates a barrier, making it more difficult for LDL to enter the artery wall.

HDL also prevents the platelets (our blood-clotting cells) from clumping together. Because a heart attack is generally the result of a cholesterol deposit with a blood clot on top, preventing clots is very important in preventing heart attacks.

The relative importance of each of these additional HDL effects is unknown, but will likely be explored in the next few years.

No matter what your lipid problem is, it is very likely that improved therapies will become available in the next few years. But it is important to remember that diet and exercise are still the cornerstones of cholesterol management. Not only do diet and exercise protect you from heart disease and stroke, they are crucial for the prevention of many other chronic illnesses. There will, however, be many cases in which diet and exercise fail to completely correct a person's lipid problem. In this situation, don't be afraid to embrace modern medicine; it may save your life.

Conclusion

I hope you have enjoyed this book. I bet you were surprised
that there is so much to say about cholesterol. But isn't this
the way it is with most fields? The more you know, the more
there is to know. When it comes to improving *your* cholesterol, I am a firm believer that the more you know, the better. After all, it is your body, and you are the person with a
cholesterol that needs improving. You deserve to know as
much as possible. If you have read this book carefully, at
this point you probably know as much (if not more) about
cholesterol as most practicing physicians.

I hope the information outlined in this book helped you
identify changes that you can make in your lifestyle. As you
make these changes, remember that you are reworking old
habits, and old habits die hard. (That's why they call them
habits!) If you slip up with your diet, exercise, or alcohol
intake—or if you smoke a cigarette—don't be too hard on
yourself. Most of all, don't give up. Carefully examine what

happened, and identify a plan to prevent it from happening again. You can do it!

Many people tell me that they feel like a failure if they require a cholesterol-altering medication. However, if you have heart disease (where cholesterol goals are very strict) or you have a genetic cholesterol abnormality, cholesterol-altering medications are likely to be necessary. If you need a medication, please take it faithfully. It may save your life.

For people with cholesterol disorders, the future has never looked so good. We know more than ever about diet, exercise, and nutritional supplements. And the cholesterol-lowering medications we have are good and promise to get better. Please use the information you have learned in this book and decide today to live a long and happy life.

Glossary

Aerobic exercise Exercise in which the muscles utilize oxygen (aerobic means "with oxygen") to burn both sugar and body fat. Examples include walking, running, swimming, biking, and skiing.

Anaerobic exercise Exercise that is performed in short intense bursts and does not utilize oxygen. Examples include weight lifting and sprinting.

Angina pectoris Chest pain or pressure resulting from insufficient blood flow (and oxygen delivery) to the heart muscle—typically, the result of blockages within the coronary arteries. In some people, angina is felt as arm, jaw, or neck pain.

Angioplasty See **Coronary artery balloon angioplasty**.

Antioxidant A dietary supplement or medication that prevents LDL cholesterol (the bad cholesterol) from becoming oxidized. Studies indicate that oxidized LDL cholesterol is a major component of plaque within the artery wall. Examples of antioxidants include estrogen and Vitamins E and C. Although these agents appear to prevent oxidation of LDL cholesterol, their role in cardiac risk reduction is uncertain at this time.

Arrhythmia An electrical disturbance in the heart rhythm, which is often the result of underlying coronary artery disease.

Atherosclerosis A disease process that begins in childhood, characterized by the gradual buildup of plaque within the artery wall. Cholesterol is a major component of the plaque. When a plaque becomes unstable, it can rupture. A blood clot may form at the site of rupture, leading to a complete blockage of the artery. When this occurs in a heart artery, the result may be a heart attack or angina.

Benecol A plant stanol margarine. When two tablespoons of Benecol are used per day, LDL cholesterol can be expected to fall approximately 14 percent. In our clinic, we favor the use of Benecol Light, which has fewer calories and less fat than the regular Benecol.

Beta-blocker A medication used for the treatment of high blood pressure or angina (chest pain or pressure). Beta-blockers reduce the work of the heart by slowing the heart rate. Side effects include fatigue, cold hands and feet, vivid dreams, and sometimes impotence. Beta-blockers can also result in an increase in triglycerides and a reduction in HDL cholesterol (the protective cholesterol).

Bypass See **Coronary artery bypass grafting**.

Carbohydrate A sugar or starch. One gram of carbohydrate contains four calories.

Cardiac Pertaining to the heart.

Cardiac catheterization See **Coronary angiography.**

Cardiac rehabilitation program A three-times-weekly, medically supervised exercise program attended by people with cardiac disease. Such programs also generally include classes on smoking cessation, diet, and stress reduction.

Cardiac risk factors Aspects of a person's life that predispose him or her to the development of cardiac disease. These include elevated LDL cholesterol (the bad cholesterol), depressed HDL cholesterol (the good cholesterol), elevated triglycerides, smoking, diabetes, a family history of heart disease, obesity, sedentary lifestyle, high blood pressure, an elevated lipoprotein(a) level, an elevated homocysteine level, an elevated C-reactive protein level, and being a male over the age of 45 or being a postmenopausal female.

Catheterization See **Coronary angiography.**

Cholesterol A white, waxy substance found only in products of animal origin, including eggs, meat, milk, cheese, and ice cream. Cholesterol is also produced by our cells (most notably, by our liver cells). Small amounts of cholesterol are necessary to make cell membranes and hormones.

Cholestin Red yeast fermented on rice. When a total of 2,400 mg of Cholestin are taken per day, a 20 percent reduction in LDL cholesterol can be expected.

Coronary angiography A procedure in which dye is injected into the coronary arteries via a flexible catheter (a thin, hollow plastic tube) to determine if these arteries have significant blockages.

Coronary artery An artery that supplies blood and oxygen to the heart muscle. Coronary arteries arise from the aorta. The major coronary arteries include the right coronary artery and the left main artery, which quickly divides into the circumflex and left anterior descending arteries.

Coronary artery balloon angioplasty A procedure in which a thin catheter containing an inflatable balloon is used to open a blocked coronary artery. Metal stents (metal springs, much like those found in a pen) are frequently placed at the angioplasty site to prevent recurring blockage.

Coronary artery bypass grafting Open-heart surgery in which a leg vein (saphenous vein) or breast artery (mammary artery) is used to connect the aorta with a coronary artery just beyond a cholesterol blockage. Over the past few years, newer and less invasive techniques have been developed to allow coronary artery bypass grafting to be performed without the need for a large chest-wall incision.

Coronary artery disease (CAD) A progressive disorder caused by blockages within the coronary arteries. Aftereffects of this disease include angina pectoris, heart attack, and sudden cardiac death. Individuals with coronary artery disease may require coronary artery balloon angioplasty or coronary artery bypass grafting.

Coronary-care unit An intensive-care unit within a hospital in which cardiac patients receive specialized monitoring and care. Such units are equipped with defibrillators, respirators, and other life-sustaining equipment.

Diabetes A disease characterized by a fasting blood sugar of greater than 126 mg/dl when measured on several different occasions. Having diabetes dramatically increases a person's risk of developing cardiac disease.

Electrocardiogram Often referred to as an EKG or ECG, an electrocardiogram is a painless procedure in which electrodes are placed on the chest wall, arms, and legs and used to monitor electrical impulses as they pass through the heart muscle, controlling its activity. In some situations, the EKG is combined with exercise (a stress test). This is done to detect electrical disturbances that might not be evident at rest.

Endothelium The inner lining of an artery.

Estrogen A female sex hormone produced by the ovaries. After menopause the production of estrogen is drastically reduced. Although estrogen deficiency is believed to be one of the major causes for the increase in cardiac events in postmenopausal women, at this writing estrogen replacement therapy has not been shown to decrease cardiac risk.

Familial combined hyperlipidemia (FCH) A genetic cholesterol disorder. Afflicted persons may have an elevated LDL cholesterol (bad cholesterol) level, an elevated triglyceride level, or elevations of both these lipoproteins. Regardless of the specific cholesterol abnormality, people with FCH are at high risk for the development of premature cardiac disease. FCH is the most common inherited cholesterol abnormality, affecting roughly one person in every 100 in the United States.

Familial hypercholesterolemia (FH) A genetic cholesterol disorder that prevents affected individuals from processing LDL cholesterol (the bad cholesterol) properly. Persons who have inherited two genes for this disorder may have a total cholesterol level of up to 1000 mg/dl and will often have their first heart attack in the first decade of their life.

Those who have inherited only one gene for the disorder typically have a cholesterol level of 300 to 500 mg/dl. If left untreated, those who suffer from the condition can expect a heart attack in middle age.

Highly effective drug therapies are available for people who have inherited a single gene for this disorder. Therapy for the rare person who has inherited two genes for FH consists primarily of LDL apheresis.

Fiber Roughage, or material found in plants and vegetables that is resistant to digestion. Fiber may be either water-soluble or water-insoluble. Water-soluble fiber is found in fruits, beans, oatmeal, and legumes. This type of fiber helps to reduce cholesterol level. Water-insoluble fiber, found mostly in grains and vegetables, may help prevent constipation.

Fish oil Oils found in fish and other marine life. The major fish oils are eicosapentenoic acid (EPA) and docosahexenoic acid (DHA). These are also known as omega-3 fatty acids). In high doses, fish oils have been shown to lower triglycerides. At low doses, fish oils appear to reduce the risk of sudden cardiac death.

Flaxseed Ground flaxseed is an excellent plant source of the omega-3 fatty acid alpha-linolenic acid (ALA). It is also rich in fiber and plant lignans. These ingredients provide ground flaxseed with its cholesterol-lowering effect.

Folic Acid A dietary constituent found in foods such as lima beans, broccoli, spinach, asparagus, potatoes, whole-wheat bread, and dried beans. Folic acid is necessary for homocysteine metabolism. Elevated homocysteine levels are a risk factor for the development of heart disease.

Guggulipid A resin or sap from *Commiphora mukul* (the mukul myrrh tree). The active ingredients in guggulipid are two plant steroids, which may reduce LDL cholesterol by about 12 percent and triglycerides by as much as 15 percent.

Heart attack See **Myocardial Infarction.**

High-density lipoprotein cholesterol (HDL-C) Often referred to as the "good" cholesterol, high levels of this lipoprotein protect against heart disease through a process called reverse cholesterol transport.

HMG CoA reductase inhibitor A class of cholesterol-lowering drugs that includes atorvastatin (Lipitor), simvastatin (Zocor), pravastatin (Pravachol), fluvastatin (Lescol), and lovastatin (Mevacor). This group of drugs is called the *statins*. These drugs lower LDL cholesterol dramatically. It is likely that several new statins will soon be on the market. Rosuvastatin (Crestor) is likely to be on the market in the year 2002.

Hypercholesterolemia An elevated cholesterol level.

Hypothyroidism A condition in which the thyroid gland is underactive. This condition may lead to marked triglyceride elevations. Therapy involves daily thyroid hormone replacement in the form of a pill.

LDL apheresis A procedure in which blood is removed from the body (via a needle in an arm vein), cleansed of cholesterol, and returned to the body via a needle in the opposite arm. Although this procedure can dramatically lower LDL cholesterol (by up to 70 percent), it needs to be repeated every two weeks, takes up to three hours, and is very expensive.

Lecithin A dietary supplement that does not help to lower cholesterol.

Legume Edible seeds enclosed in pods. Examples include soybeans, lima beans, peas, lentils, black beans, kidney beans, black-eyed peas, chickpeas, and cannellini beans.

Lipid profile A blood test that reports total cholesterol, triglycerides, HDL cholesterol, and LDL cholesterol.

Lipoprotein(a) An LDL-like particle with an attached protein called apoprotein(a). It is found in the bloodstream. Elevated levels of this blood lipid increase a person's risk of developing early heart disease.

Low-density lipoprotein cholesterol (LDL-C) Often referred to as the "bad" cholesterol; elevated levels of this blood fat increase the risk of developing early heart disease.

Menopause The time in a woman's life when the ovaries cease to produce the female sex hormones, estrogen and progesterone. In the United States, the average woman enters menopause at age 51. Women who smoke cigarettes generally enter menopause at an earlier age.

Monounsaturated fat The type of fat found in olive oil, canola oil, and peanut oil. When this type of fat is substituted for saturated fat, LDL cholesterol level will fall and HDL cholesterol may rise.

Myocardial infarction A heart attack. This condition develops when an area of heart muscle is deprived of oxygen. The result is cellular death and eventual scar formation.

Myositis A rare condition characterized by fever, muscle cramping, and weakness. If myositis progresses to the point where muscle-cell breakdown and kidney failure occurs, the condition is called rhabdomyolysis.

Oat bran A water-soluble fiber known to lower cholesterol.

Pectin The cholesterol-lowering, water-soluble fiber found in fruit.

Plant stanol/sterol A substance found in plants (and in the margarines Benecol and Take Control). Plant stanols and sterols prevent the absorption of dietary cholesterol. This results in as much as a 14 percent reduction in the LDL cholesterol level.

Plaque A blockage within an artery composed of cholesterol, cellular debris, and fibrous material.

Platelet A blood-clotting cell.

Polyunsaturated fat The type of fat found in corn, sunflower, and safflower oils. When this type of fat is substituted for saturated fat, both total and HDL cholesterol may fall.

Progesterone A female sex hormone produced by the ovaries. Like estrogen, progesterone ceases to be produced at menopause.

Protein An essential element of the diet that contains amino acids, carbon, hydrogen, oxygen, and nitrogen. Protein is plentiful in grains, poultry, and dairy products and can be obtained in sufficient amounts without consuming meat. Each gram of protein contains four calories.

Psyllium A cholesterol-lowering, water-soluble fiber found in products like Metamucil. Some cereals are enriched with psyllium; such cereals lower cholesterol.

Rhabdomyolysis See **Myositis.**

Saturated fat The type of fat found in butter, cheese, whole milk, ice cream, white marbling in meat, palm oil, and coconut oils. This type of fat is known to increase cholesterol levels dramatically.

Soy protein Protein found in products made from soybeans. Consumption of 24 grams of soy protein per day will result in about a 13 percent reduction in LDL cholesterol and a 10 percent reduction in triglyceride level. Good sources of soy protein include soy milk, soy nuts, soy cheeses, and soy burgers, as well as tofu and tempeh.

Stress test See **Electrocardiogram.**

Take Control A plant sterol margarine. Use of two tablespoons per day of this margarine can result in approximately a 10 percent fall in LDL cholesterol.

Tissue plasminogen activator (TPA) A clot-dissolving agent.

Trans fat The type of fat created when liquid oils (such as canola, olive, corn, or sunflower) undergo a process called hydrogenation. The resulting fat behaves much the way saturated fat does, leading to an increase in cholesterol levels. Trans fats also are known to cause the HDL cholesterol level to fall. Trans fats are abundant in deep-fried fast foods and commercially prepared baked goods.

Triglyceride One of the blood fats. Triglycerides may be made by the liver or ingested through the diet. An elevated triglyceride level appears to be a strong predictor of cardiac disease, especially in women.

Wheat bran A water-insoluble fiber that does not lower cholesterol, but may help relieve constipation.

Xanthelasma A yellowish deposit of cholesterol on the eyelid or under the eye. Its presence suggests that the cholesterol level is elevated.

Xanthoma A cholesterol deposit typically found in the tendons of the hand or ankle. Xanthomas are found in approximately 75 percent of adults with familial hypercholesterolemia.

Bibliography

Acton, S., et al. "Identification of scavenger receptor SR-BI as a high-density lipoprotein receptor." *Science* 271, 1996: 518–520.

Adler, A. J., and B. J. Holub. "Effect of garlic and fish-oil supplementation on serum lipid and lipoprotein concentrations in hypercholesterolemic men." *American Journal of Clinical Nutrition* 65, 1997: 445–450.

Anderson, J. W., et al. "Cholesterol-lowering effects of psyllium intake adjunctive to diet therapy in men and women with hypercholesterolemia: meta-analysis of eight controlled trials." *American Journal of Clinical Nutrition* 71, 2000: 472–479.

———. "Meta-analysis of the effects of soy protein intake on serum lipids." *New England Journal of Medicine* 333, 1995: 276–282.

Anderson, L. B., et al. "All-cause mortality associated with physical activity during leisure time, work, sports, and cycling to work." *Archives of Internal Medicine* 160, 2000: 1621–1628.

Arjmandi, B. H., et al. "Whole flaxseed consumption lowers serum LDL cholesterol and lipoprotein(a) concentrations in postmenopausal women." *Nutrition Research* 18, Vol. 7, 1998: 1203–1214.

Ask, E. N. "Can the sap from an Indian shrub lower cholesterol?" *Environmental Nutrition*, January 1999: 7.

Assmann, G., et al. "Familial high-density lipoprotein deficiency: Tangier disease." *The Metabolic and Molecular Bases of Inherited Disease*, C. R. Scriver, ed. New York: McGraw-Hill, 1995.

Bailey, C. *The New Fit or Fat*. Boston: Houghton Mifflin, 1991.

Bakker-Arkema, R. G., et al. "Efficacy and safety of a new HMG-CoA Reductase inhibitor, atorvastatin, in patients with hypertriglyceridemia." *Journal of the American Medical Association* 275, 1996: 128–133.

Berthold, H. K., et al. "Effect of a garlic-oil preparation on serum lipoproteins and cholesterol metabolism." *Journal of the American Medical Association* 279, 1998: 1900–1902.

Blondal, T., et al. "Nicotine nasal spray with nicotine patch for smoking cessation: randomized trial with six-year follow-up." *British Medical Journal* 318, 1999: 285–289.

"Blood Feud." *Forbes*, 22 January 2001: 67–68.

Blum, C. B. "Comparison of properties of four inhibitors of 3-hydroxy-3-methylglutaryl-coenzyme A reductase." *American Journal of Cardiology* 73, 1994: 3D–11D.

Breslow, J. L. "Familial disorders of high-density lipoprotein metabolism." *The Metabolic and Molecular Bases of Inherited Disease*, C. R. Scriver, ed. New York: McGraw-Hill, 1995.

Brody, Jane. *Jane Brody's Good Food Book: Living the High Carbohydrate Way*. Toronto: Bantam Books, 1987.

Brooks-Wilson, A., et al. "Mutations in ABC1 in Tangier disease and familial high-density lipoprotein deficiency." *Nature Genetics* 22, 1999: 336–344.

Brown, L., et al. "Cholesterol-lowering effects of dietary fiber: a meta-analysis." *American Journal of Clinical Nutrition* 69, 1999: 30–42.

Burr, M. L., et al. "Effects of changes in fat, fish, and fibre intakes on death and myocardial infarction: diet and reinfarction trial (DART)." *Lancet* 2, 1989: 757–761.

Canner, P. L., et al., for the Coronary Drug Project Research Group. "Fifteen-year mortality in Coronary Drug Project patients: long-term benefit with niacin." *American Journal of Cardiology* 8, 1986: 1245–1255.

Cholesterol Medical Technology Stock Letter 408, November 2000.

Carr, A., et al. "A syndrome of peripheral lipodystrophy, hyperlipidemia and insulin resistance in patients receiving HIV protease inhibitors." *AIDS* 12, 1998: F51–F58.

"Colesevelam (Welchol) for hypercholesterolemia." *The Medical Letter* 42, 2000: 102–103.

Compestine, Y. C. *Secrets of Fat-Free Chinese Cooking.* Garden City Park: Avery Publishing Group, 1997.

Connor, S., and W. Connor. *The New American Diet.* New York: Simon & Schuster, 1991.

Connor, W. E., and S. L. Connor. "The dietary therapy of hyperlipidemia: its important role in the prevention of heart disease." In *Handbook of Experimental Pharmacology, Vol. 109: Principles and Treatment of Lipoprotein Disorders,* G. Schettler and A. J. R. Habenicht, eds. Berlin: Springer-Verlag, 1994.

Connor, W., et al. "The plasma lipids, lipoproteins, and diet of the Tarahumara Indians." *The American Journal of Clinical Nutrition* 31, 1978: 1131–1142.

Crane, K. W. "Nature's best medicines." *Prevention,* October 1997, 99–100.

Davidson, M. H., et al. "Colesevelam hydrochloride (cholestagel). A new, potent bile acid sequestrant associated with a low incidence of gastrointestinal side effects." *The Archives of Internal Medicine* 159, 1999: 1893–1899.

———. "ZD4522 is superior to atorvastatin in decreasing low density lipoprotein cholesterol and increasing high density lipoprotein cholesterol in patients with Type IIa or IIb hypercholesterolemia." Abstract presented at American College of Cardiology meeting: Orlando, Florida: March 2001.

Dengel, D. R., et al. "Comparable effects of diet and exercise on body composition and lipoproteins in older men." *Medicine, Science, Sports and Exercise* 26, 1994: 1307–1315.

Denke, M. A., et al. "Individual cholesterol variation in response to a margarine- or butter-based diet: a study in families." *Journal of the American Medical Association* 284, 2000: 2740–2747.

Eder, A. F., and D. J. Rader. "LDL apheresis for severe refractory dyslipidemia." *Today's Therapeutic Trends* 14, 1996: 165–179.

Fagerstrom, K. O. "Measuring degree of physical dependence to tobacco smoking with reference to individualization of treatment." *Addictive Behaviors* 3, 1978: 235–241.

Farquhar, J. W., et al. "The effect of beta-sitosterol on the serum lipids in young men with arteriosclerotic heart disease." *Circulation* 14, 1956: 77–82.

Fiore, M. C., S. S. Smith, and D. E. Jorenby, et al. "The effectiveness of the nicotine patch for smoking cessation." *Journal of the American Medical Association* 271, 1994: 1940–1947.

Fraser, G. E., et al. "The Adventist health study: A possible protective effect of nut consumption on risk of coronary heart disease." *Archives of Internal Medicine* 152, 1992: 1416–1424.

Frick, M. H., et al. "Helsinki heart study: primary-prevention trial with gemfibrozil in middle-aged men with dyslipidemia." *New England Journal of Medicine* 317, 1987: 1237–1245.

Garrison, R. J., et al. "Cigarette smoking and HDL cholesterol: The Framingham Offspring study." *Atherosclerosis* 30, 1978: 17–25.

Glore, S. R., et al. "Soluble fiber and serum lipids: a literature review." *Journal of the American Dietetic Association* 94, 1994: 425–436.

Goldstein, J., et al. "Familial hypercholesterolemia." In *The Metabolic and Molecular Bases of Inherited Disease*, C. R. Scriver, ed. New York: McGraw-Hill, 1995.

Goor, R., and Nancy Goor. *Eater's Choice*. Boston: Houghton Mifflin, 1989.

Grupo Italiano per lo Studio della Sopravivenza nell'Infarto miocardico. "Dietary supplementation with n-3 polyunsaturated fatty acids and vitamin E after myocardial infarction: results of the GISSI-Prevenzione Study." *Lancet* 354, 1999: 447–455.

Hallikainen, M. A., et al. "Effects of two low-fat stanol ester-containing margarines on serum cholesterol concentrations as part of a low-fat diet in hypercholesterolemic subjects." *American Journal of Clinical Nutrition* 69, 1999: 403–410.

Havel, R. J. "Dietary supplement or drug? The case of Cholestin." *American Journal of Clinical Nutrition* 69, 1999: 175–176.

Heber, D., et al. "Cholesterol lowering effects of a proprietary Chinese red-yeast rice dietary supplement." *American Journal of Clinical Nutrition* 69, 1999: 231–236.

Henkin, Y., et al. "Secondary dyslipidemia: inadvertent effects of drugs in clinical practice." *Journal of the American Medical Association* 267, 1992: 961–968.

Henry, K., et al. "Atorvastatin and gemfibrozil for protease-inhibitor–related lipid abnormalities." *Lancet* 352, 1998: 1031–1032.

Holloszy, J. O. "Effects of a six-month program of endurance exercise on serum lipids of middle-aged men." *American Journal of Cardiology* 14, 1964: 753–760.

Jorenby, D. E., and S. J. Leischow. "A controlled trial of sustained-release bupropion, a nicotine patch, or both for smoking cessation." *The New England Journal of Medicine* 340, 1999: 685–691.

Kane, J., and R. J. Havel. "Disorders of the biogenesis and secretion of lipoproteins containing the B apolipoproteins." In *The Metabolic and Molecular Bases of Inherited Disease,* C. R. Scriver, ed. New York: McGraw-Hill, 1995.

Kestin, M., et al. "N-3 fatty acids of marine origin lower systolic blood pressure and triglycerides but raise LDL cholesterol compared with N-3 and N-6 fatty acids from plants." *American Journal of Clinical Nutrition* 51, 1990: 1028–1034.

Kosoglou, T., et al. "Pharmacodynamic interaction between the new selective cholesterol absorption inhibitor ezetimibe and atorvastatin." Abstract presented at American College of Cardiology meeting: Orlando, Florida: March 2001.

Krauss, R. M., et al. "AHA Dietary Guidelines: Revision 2000. A statement for healthcare professionals from the nutrition committee of the American Heart Association." *Circulation* 102, 2000: 2284–2299.

Kwiterovich, P. *Beyond Cholesterol*. Baltimore: The Johns University Press, 1989.

LaRosa, J. C. "Combinations of drugs in lipid-lowering therapy." *American Journal of Medicine* 96, 1994: 399–400.

Lavie, C. J., and R. V. Milani. "Effects of nonpharmacologic therapy with cardiac rehabilitation and exercise training in patients with low levels of high-density lipoprotein cholesterol." *The American Journal of Cardiology* 78, 1996: 1286–1289.

———. "Factors predicting improvements in lipid values following cardiac rehabilitation and exercise training." *Archives of Internal Medicine* 153, 1993: 982–988.

Lee, I. M., et al. "Physical activity and coronary heart disease risk in men: does the duration of exercise episodes predict risk?" *Circulation* 102, 2000: 981–986.

Lees, A. M., et al. "Plant sterols as cholesterol-lowering agents: clinical trials in patients with hypercholesterolemia and studies of sterol balance." *Atherosclerosis* 28, Vol. 3, 1977: 325–328.

The Lipid Research Clinics Coronary Primary Prevention Trial Results. "Reduction in the incidence of coronary heart disease." *Journal of the American Medical Association* 251, 1984: 351–364.

———. "The relationship in incidence of coronary heart disease to cholesterol lowering." *Journal of the American Medical Association* 251, 1984: 365–374.

Maher, V. M., et al. "Effects of lowering elevated LDL cholesterol on the cardiovascular risk of lipoprotein (a)." *Journal of the American Medical Association* 274, 1995: 1771–1774.

Masley, S. C., et al. "Dietary therapy for preventing and treating coronary artery disease." *American Family Physician* 57, 1998: 1299–1306.

Mateljan, G. *Cooking Without Fat.* New York: Villard, 1996.

Mattson, F. H., et al. "Optimizing the effect of plant sterols on cholesterol absorption in man." *American Journal of Clinical Nutrition* 35, Vol. 4, 1982: 697–700.

McGowan, M. P. *Heart Fitness for Life.* New York: Oxford University Press, 1997.

Miettinen, T. A., et al. "Reduction of serum cholesterol with Sitostanol-ester margarine in a mildly hyper-cholesterolemic population." *New England Journal of Medicine* 333, 1995: 1308–1312.

Morgan, J. M., and D. M. Capuzzi. "Combination therapy in the control of combined hyperlipidemia: the role of extended-release niacin." *Cardiovascular Reviews & Reports* 21, 2000: 1–7.

Morgan, J. M., et al. "Treatment effect of Niaspan, a controlled-release niacin, in patients with hyper-cholesterolemia: a placebo-controlled trial." *Journal of Cardiovascular Pharmacology and Therapeutics* 1, 1996: 195–202.

Ockene, J. K. "Smoking interventions: a behavioral, educational, and pharmacological perspective." In *Prevention of Coronary Heart Disease*, I. S. Ockene and J. K. Ockene, eds. Boston: Little, Brown, 1992.

Olson, B. H., et al. "Psyllium-enriched cereals lower blood total cholesterol and LDL cholesterol, but not HDL cholesterol, in hypercholesterolemic adults: results of a meta-analysis." *Journal of Nutrition* 127, 1997: 1973–1980.

Ottariano, S. *Medicinal Herbal Therapy: A Pharmacist's Viewpoint.* Portsmouth: Nicoli Fields Publishing, 1999.

Paffenbarger, R. S., Jr., et al. "The association of changes in physical-activity level and other lifestyle characteristics with mortality among men." *New England Journal of Medicine* 328, 1993: 538–545.

Paoletti, R., et al. "ZD4522 is superior to pravastatin and simvastatin in reducing low density lipoprotein cholesterol, enabling more hypercholesterolemic patients to achieve target low density lipoprotein cholesterol guidelines." Abstract presented at American College of Cardiology meeting: Orlando, Florida: March 2001.

Patrick, M. A., et al. "CAVEAT: a randomized, double-blind, parallel group evaluation of cerivastatin 0.4 mg and 0.8 mg compared to atorvastatin 10 mg and 20 mg once daily in patients with combined (type IIb) dyslipidemia." *The British Journal of Cardiology* 7, 2000: 780–786.

Pearson, T. A. "The lipid treatment assessment project (L-TAP): a multicenter survey to evaluate the percentages of dyslipidemic patients receiving lipid-lowering therapy and achieving low-density lipoprotein cholesterol goals." *Archives of Internal Medicine* 160, 459–467.

Piscatella, J. *Controlling Your Fat Tooth.* New York: Workman Publishing Company, 1991.

Pitt, B., et al. "Aggressive lipid-lowering therapy compared with angioplasty in stable coronary artery disease." *New England Journal of Medicine* 341, 1999: 70–76.

Potter, S. M., et al. "Depression of plasma cholesterol in men by consumption of baked products containing soy protein." *American Journal of Clinical Nutrition* 58, 1993: 501–506.

Prasad, K. "Dietary flaxseed in prevention of hyper-cholesterolemic atherosclerosis." *Atherosclerosis* 132, 1997: 69–76.

Rippe, J,. et al. "A multi-center, self-controlled study of Cholestin™ in subjects with elevated cholesterol." American Heart Association: 39th Annual Conference on Cardiovascular Disease Epidemiology and Prevention. Orlando, Florida: March 24–27, 1999.

Sabaté, J., et al. "Effects of walnuts on serum lipid levels and blood pressure in normal men." *New England Journal of Medicine* 328, 1993: 603–607.

Scanu, A. M., et al. "Lipoprotein(a) and atherosclerosis." *Annals of Internal Medicine* 115, 1991: 209–218.

Schuler, G. H. "Regular physical exercise and low-fat diet: effects on progression of coronary artery disease." *Circulation* 86, 1992: 1–11.

Schwartz, G. G., et al. "The myocardial ischemia reduction with aggressive cholesterol lowering (MIRACL) study." Presented at the American Heart Association

73rd Scientific Sessions, New Orleans, Louisiana: November 2000.

Singh, R. B., et al. "Hypolipidemic and antioxidant effects of *Commiphora mukul* as an adjunct to dietary therapy in patients with hypercholesterolemia." *Cardiovascular Drugs and Therapeutics* 8, 1994: 659–664.

Singh, V., et al. "Stimulation of low-density lipoprotein receptor activity in liver membrane of guggulsterone-treated rats." *Pharmacological Research* 22, 1990: 37–44.

Sirtori, C. R., et al. "Soy and cholesterol reduction: clinical experience." *Journal of Nutrition* 125, 1995: Supplement 598S–605S

———. "Soybean-protein diet in the treatment of type II hyperlipoproteinaemia." *Lancet* 1, 1977: 275–277.

Stein, E., et al. "ZD4522 (Rosuvastatin) compared with diet and maximal lipid therapy in patients with heterozygous familial hypercholesterolemia." Abstract presented at American College of Cardiology meeting: Orlando, Florida: March 2001.

———. "ZD4522 is superior to atorvastatin in the treatment of patients with heterozygous familial hypercholesterolemia." Abstract presented at American College of Cardiology meeting, Orlando: Florida: March 2001.

Stevinson, C., et al. "Garlic for treating hypercholesterolemia." *Annals of Internal Medicine* 133, 2000: 420–429.

Stone, N. J. "Fish consumption, fish oil, lipids, and coronary heart disease." *Circulation* 94, 1996: 2337–2340.

Summary of the second report of the National Cholesterol Education Program (NCEP) Expert Panel on
detection, evaluation, and treatment of high blood
cholesterol in adults (Adult Treatment Panel II).
Journal of the American Medical Association 269, 1993:
3015–3023.

Tyler, V. E. *Herbs of Choice: The Therapeutic Use of Phytomedici-
nals.* Binghamton: Hawthorn Press, Inc., 1994.

U.S. Department of Health and Human Services. *Physical
Activity and Health: A Report of the Surgeon General.*
Atlanta, GA: Centers for Disease Control and
Prevention, National Center for Chronic Disease
Prevention and Health Promotion, 1996.

Vegh-Dunn, A. "Incorporating soy protein into a low-fat
low-cholesterol diet." *Cleveland Clinic Journal of
Medicine* 67, 2000: 767–772.

Verrillo, A., et al. "Soybean protein diets in the management of type II hyperlipoproteinaemia." *Atherosclerosis* 54, 1985: 321–331.

Wang, J,. et al. "Multicenter clinical trial of the serum
lipid–lowering effects of monascus purpureus (red
yeast) rice preparation from traditional Chinese
medicine." *Current Therapeutic Research* 58, 1997:
964–978.

Ward, A., et al. "Exercise and exercise intervention." In
Prevention of Coronary Heart Disease, I. S. Ockene and
J. K. Ockene, eds. Boston: Little, Brown, 1992.

Warshafsky, S., et al. "Effect of garlic on total serum
cholesterol: a meta-analysis." *Annals of Internal
Medicine* 119, 1993: 599–600.

Webb, D. "Forgotten cholesterol cure uncovered—
    phytosterols, first tested in the '50s, are finally
    getting the attention they deserve." *Prevention*,
    December 2000, 65–66.

Wood, P. D., et al. "Increased exercise level and plasma
    lipoprotein concentrations: a one-year randomized
    controlled study in sedentary middle-aged men."
    Metabolism 32, 1983: 31–39.

Writing Group for the PEPI Trial. "Effects of estrogen of
    estrogen/progestin regimens on heart disease risk
    factors in postmenopausal women." *Journal of the
    American Medical Association* 273, 1995: 199–208.

Young, S. G., and C. J. Fielding. "The ABCs of Choles-
    terol Efflux." *Nature Genetics* 22, 1999: 336–344.

Zambon, D., et al. "Substituting walnuts for monounsatu-
    rated fat improves the serum lipid profile of hyper-
    cholesterolemic men and women." *Annals of Internal
    Medicine* 132, 2000: 538–546.

Zeni, A. I., et al. "Energy expenditures with indoor exer-
    cise machines." *Journal of the American Medical Associa-
    tion* 275, 1996: 1424–1427.

Index